2

D0905162

SEX, SHAME, AND VIOLENCE

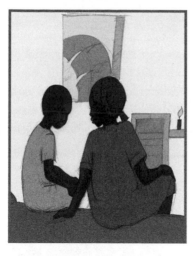

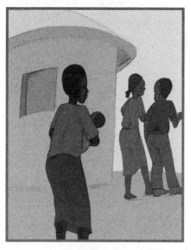

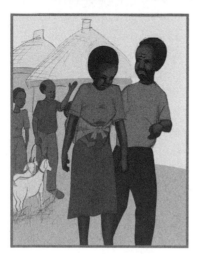

SEX, SHAME,
AND VIOLENCE

A Revolutionary Practice
of Public Storytelling
in Poor Communities

KATHLEEN CASH

I.C.C. LIBRARY

Vanderbilt University Press
NASHVILLE

RA
418.5
.C375
2016

© 2016 by Kathleen Cash
All rights reserved
Published 2016 by Vanderbilt University Press
Nashville, Tennessee 37235
First printing 2016

This book is printed on acid-free paper.
Manufactured in the United States of America

Frontispiece: Images from *Agnes*, a narrative
used in the Ugandan project.

Library of Congress Cataloging-in-Publication Data on file

LC control number 2014030777
LC classification number RA418.5.P6
Dewey class number 362.1086'942—dc23

ISBN 978-0-8265-2050-0 (hardcover)
ISBN 978-0-8265-2051-7 (paperback)
ISBN 978-0-8265-2052-4 (ebook)

To Shama, Sophie, and Rose,

and to my parents, Isabel and Irv—

for their generosity in immeasurable ways

6/17 YBP 29.95

Contents

Acknowledgments

I am very grateful to the hundreds of people who willingly became involved in various aspects of the eight projects that are the basis of this book, as research respondents, participants, and even families or friends of participants. For some, this took many hours of their time, in sometimes blistering heat, without material compensation, which demonstrated a belief that this project had something of value to offer them. I do not know the names of all these people, but I have images of them and recollections of their stories.

Over fifteen hundred people have been instrumental in the development and field-testing of these projects. These people have been administrators, researchers, translators, artists, facilitators, and evaluators. Though there are too many to acknowledge, these are a few to whom I am particularly grateful.

From the Thai project: At International Center for Research for Women (ICRW, *www.icrw.org*), an organization conducting research dedicated to empowering women, director Geeta Rao Gupta, and staff Ellen Weiss and Daniel Whelan. At Chiang Mai University, Deans Kasem Wattananchai and Jaratbhan Sanguansermsri; project staff Bupa Anasuchatkul, Porntip Chuamanochan, and Rachanee Sriornsri; translators Srivilai Dorkchan and Narin Kaewmeesri; and artists Wattana Wattanapun and Nat Tamrongpittayanan.

From the Bangladeshi project: At BRAC (*www.brac.net*), an organization dedicated to alleviating poverty, director Fazel Hassan Abed; staff A. Mushtaque R. Chowdhury, Sadia Chowdhury, and Kanis Fatima; and project staff Hashima-E-Nasreen. At International Centre for Diarrhoeal Disease Research, Bangladesh (ICDDR,B), an international health research institution, director Abbas Bhuiya and project staff Ayesha Aziz.

From the Haitian projects: Under the auspices of Fonkoze (*www.fonkoze.org*), Haiti's largest microfinance institution that works to provide financial and non-financial services for poor Haitian women, director Anne Hastings; project staff Jean Giny Casseus, Dominique, Jean Reynolds Imera, Patrice Fougan, Nicolas Ledoux, Megan Affronti, and Jennifer Joyce; facilitators Micheline Fleurimond, Lianne Joseph, Darline Malvoisin, Inofie Malvoisin, Juline Salomon, and Molienne Samuelle. At Hospital Albert Schweitzer, director Henry Perry; staff Rubin Petit, Gabriel Joseph, Alex Smith, Johann Preval, and Eric E. N. Jean; artists Albert Coussaint and Bon-Aime Johnson. From Beyond Borders (*beyondborders.net*), a nonprofit organization that works to end child slavery and violence toward women and girls, director David Diggs and project staff Myriam Narcisse, Freda Catheus, Huegel Mesidor, Andrea Pierre, Abelard Xavier, Adjanie Barthelemy, Johnny Estor, Samson Joseph, Edith Philistin, Anunondieu Jean, Reginal Jules, Antonio Presume, and Wilfaut Louis. At Matewan Community School, staff Ezner Angervil, Chris Lowe, Abner Sauveur, Benaja Antoine, Edvard Guilloteau, Emmanuel Jean, and Aunondieu Jean; translators Nadine Bellile, Ron Bluntschli, Daniel Cadet, Anna Ferdinand, Paula Hyppolite, Pierre Minn, Giscard Nazon, Tessa Richardson, Carla Bluntschli, Pierre Francillon, Frantz Henoch, Alcenat Honorat, Altidor Josue, Anne McConnell, Rodye Paquiot, Landsy Pierre, Lisa Regnier, and Geto Sainristil; artists Vady Confident, Stanley Roijude, Marco Saint Juste, Keytia, Junior Sylvaince, Ludger Bastien, Eder Romeus, Jean Louis Wisly, and Marcia Kent.

From the Latino and African American projects in Los Angeles: At Common Ground (*commongroundhiv.org*), an HIV and AIDS counseling and community center, director Jane Adams and project staff Danny Getzoff, David Kanouse, and Effraim Talavera. From the Latino project, artists Marcelo Bienevedes, Angel Garcia, Michael Docherty, Cindy Segura, and Justin Yparraguirre; facilitators Maurilia Bravo and Concepcion Rechtszaj; and the staffs of Bienstar, the Pasedena Job Center, IDEPSCA, Upward Bound House (specifically Tracy Woodbury), the Virginia Avenue Recreation Center, and Olympic High School. From the African American project, project staff Patricia "Sugar" Witherspoon, Brigitte Edwards, Sandra Cannon, and Gloria Munoz; artists Sidney James, Michael Docherty, and Carlos Juzang; consultant Hendrik Marias; and the staffs of Help the People Foundation, Clare Foundation, Sober Living, the women of His Sheltering Arms (especially Ms. Lillian Jefferies), and the men of Avalon Carter (especially Mr. D. Christenson).

From the Ugandan project: The Fulbright Foundation; the staffs of the Center for Domestic Violence and Raising Voices (*www.raisingvoices.org*), the Good Hope Foundation for Rural Development and Action Aid; artists Anjang Daniel, Ayena Patrick, Ojok Robert, Patrick Paul Kiwanuka, Marcia Kent, Angel Garcia, Jessica Cheng, Amber Helms, Sarah Gibbons, Adam Cohen, Catlin Buckley, and Janine Williams; translators Alex Ocen and Ayena Patrick. From the Lira field test, the women and men of the Starch Factory Health Care Group, the Arikino Sunday Group, the Woro Mite Group, Hosanna Vocational School, the Acake Women's Group, and Canyelo Group; facilitators Awio Dorcus, Otim Ivan, Susan Ekwar, Luci Okello, Agnes Ayo, Okabo Yeko, Odong Haggai, Okello Alfred, and Kamoga Doreen. From the Pader field test, at Concern Worldwide (*www.concern.net*), a nongovernmental international organization that works to alleviate poverty in the world's poorest countries, the directors Carol Morgan and Mary O'Neill and staff Simon Foster, Indrani Mukerjee Chris Oyua, and John Okello. From Women and Rural Development Network (Worudet), an organization dedicated to ending social injustices such as gender-based violence, director Betty Akullo and facilitators

Lam Bosco, Ocan Thomas, Atimango Florence, Banya George, Omony Edwin, Okeny John, Too-lit Bosco, Akera Valentino, Angom Duculina, Lalam Sabina, Oyella Christina, Alimo Filder, Lajara Lillian, Labongo Vento, Moro Augustina, Adiyo Polline, and Olango Samuel.

Over the years developing eight programs, I worked with people who offered support in multiple ways and with whom I have had long-lasting friendships. In Thailand, I was fortunate to have had two mentors, Ousa Thanakatul and Sirmsree Chaisorn. I am indebted to the exceptional people who went far beyond the expected as researchers, trainers, translators, advisors, and artists: Wantana Busayawong in the Thai project; Sonia Lee, Coleen Hedgelin, and Steve Werlin in the Haitian projects; Sharful "Bobby" Khan in the Bangladeshi project; Diana Andrade and Carlos Bermudez in the Latino project; Naimah Daaood and Precious Stallworth in the African American project; Sophie Adong and Omony Bosco in the Ugandan project; and Wes Casto, a graphic artist who worked on multiple projects.

Then there are those people without whose belief in my work, I would not have been able to begin and continue—people who have truly "stayed the course." I am indebted to Bill Resnick and Ruth Messenger who showed me continuous support in the magnanimity of their deeds and their character. I am very grateful to and in awe of Anne Hastings, one of the founders of Fonkoze, who gave me access to the resources of that amazing microfinance organization in order to develop three projects. Fonkoze, together with Beyond Borders, under the thoughtful leadership of David Diggs, allowed me to develop my most beloved project, the children's rights program. Special thanks to Shana Swiss, Chris Lowe, Barbie Lazarus, Carol Jenkins, and Regina Charon, with whom I shared conversations about our common beliefs; to Jessica Cheng, Colleen Hedgelin, Vinh-Kim Nguyen, Karen Manzo, and Vivian Gornick, who read my manuscript and gave me helpful suggestions.

Over many years, there are some who have been my most ardent advocates: Ioanna Trivilas, with her perspicacity, courage and caring; Diana Andrade, with her good-heartedness and resourcefulness; friends in Morgantown, Mt. Morris, Los Angeles, Stephentown, Boston, Montague, Baltimore, Laramie, New York, Milwaukee, Ames, and elsewhere—thank you all.

Judith Vichniac, the director of the Radcliffe Institute Fellowship Program, and the Hdry Foundation gave me the backing and impetus to begin this book. Geoffrey Fuller's incisive literary talents led me to the form this book finally took. Elissa Hoffman graciously and insightfully edited my manuscript. I was very fortunate to have met the Vanderbilt University Press Director, Michael Ames, who believed in my work enough to keep our conversation going through a complete revision of my manuscript. I appreciate the small village it took at Vanderbilt to put this book together, specifically Joell Smith-Borne, Dariel Mayer, Debbie Berman, Betsy Phillips, Jenna Phillips, and Silvia Benvenuto.

My sister and my brother, Ellen and Richard, have been willing, constant, and good advisors from our early beginnings. My husband, John, has generously helped me pursue my beliefs, which meant that I could leave home with a clear conscience and trust that all would be well. My daughters, Shama and Sophie, have given me invaluable homegrown advice, perceptivity, exceptional humor, and confidence. Because of all of you, for your kindness and commitment, I have been very fortunate indeed. Thank you.

Foreword

Brigitte sells coffee and hot chocolate every morning on a street corner in Anse à Galets, the one small city on La Gonâve, an island off the coast of Haiti. For less than a quarter, her customers can start their day with a hot drink and a roll. She has benches that she puts out for her clients where they sit and chat while they drink. She counts on her business to support herself and the children who still live at home with her, and the business counts on small loans that she gets from Fonkoze, Haiti's largest microfinance institution.

When Brigitte learned that her credit center would offer a class in sexual and reproductive health, she signed up right away. At sixty, Brigitte was no longer sexually active, but as a single mother of seven children ages twenty-three to thirty-five, she was surrounded by young people she worried about.

From the very beginning of the class, she was excited to discover that when she would take home the books that the class used, her children and grandchildren would come listen to the stories and read along with her. Soon they were borrowing the books and reading them on their own. And not long after that, her neighbors started sharing the books as well.

Bringing the books to work with her in the morning was just the next logical step. "I want to share information about how to protect yourself with everyone I know," she explained. Soon the topic of many of her customers' early morning conversations was reproductive health.

For Brigitte, sharing the books presented one way for her to help her family and friends look after their own health. "The books," she said, "help you understand how to avoid diseases that are really serious." And the more Brigitte shared the books, the more interest she discovered in the stories and in the themes that they raise. "Young men, older men, young women, older women: everyone gets interested in the stories and in the information the books provide." Reading the stories has given Brigitte and those around her a way to think about and talk about the most urgent issues in their own sexual lives.

Since it was founded with a mission to enable Haiti's poor to participate in their own nation's development, Fonkoze has sought to help its members—mostly poor women who live in the countryside—build the skills, assets, and capacities that they need to take on new roles in their families and communities. Its credit programs are designed to both build and depend upon solidarity among borrowers, and the education programs that support its loans are organized to develop leadership. Seen in this light, Brigitte appears as a remarkable success: a coffee merchant who has turned herself into a community educator, an agent of change.

But it is not just any educational program that could have helped Brigitte make such a dramatic transformation, and that is why we are so excited about Kathy Cash's work and about this book which explains it. Brigitte's transformation depended on two critical aspects of Kathy's work.

On the one hand, her program brings people like Brigitte into contact with stories that reflect the lives they lead. The characters they meet in the stories are like people around them. Their problems, their outlooks, even the words they use are familiar. Program participants feel as though they know the people they read about and discuss and the difficulties those people face.

On the other hand, the process that Kathy has designed for use with the stories encourages participants to turn themselves into a community of learners and then encourages them to reflect together upon the issues that the stories raise, and to do much more as well. Her programs are not about sharing information—though they are filled with good information; much less are they about preaching someone's predetermined responses to the serious questions that they raise. For Kathy, education is conversation. Participants in her programs imagine themselves as actors who are faced with serious problems, and they then take on and rewrite the roles the stories present. They create solutions and practice using the solutions, all within the fun and safe environment that the programs create.

Creating her programs is not simple. That is why we have long been hoping for this book. In it, Kathy shares both the thinking that her programs are built on and the process she uses to create the stories that the programs depend on. It is part how-to manual, part theoretical treatise, and part impassioned defense of the power of conversations to change communities and the lives lived within them.

We remember when Kathy first came to us at Fonkoze, recommended by one of our board members. We wanted a program that would transform peoples' lives. Our commitment and the commitment of our founder, Father Joseph Philippe, to liberation theology meant that any program we would get behind would have to help members learn to study their own reality critically. Kathy convinced us that her methods would help us to empower our borrowers. It would help them build their self-confidence and become leaders in their communities. They would become capable of addressing the problems they face in their lives at home and in their communities. Her methods consist of three main parts: the first is conducting ethnographic research; the second is creating the stories that become the subject matter of the class; and the third is what she calls the practice of public engagement. This is how she structures what happens in the classroom when participants hear or read a story and then reflect upon it, discuss it in depth, take on the roles of the characters in the story, and *practice* being part of the conversations raised by the story in the *presence of others*. New stories are created, new endings are practiced, and a change occurs in the participants, sometimes almost miraculously.

The result was that we welcomed her into the Fonkoze Family and gave her the freedom she needed to do her magic. She trained people from the countryside of Haiti to undertake ethnographic research by becoming interviewers who know how to conduct friendly and unhurried interviews with people from their same rural culture. Many of those interviewers are still part of Fonkoze today—some thirteen years later.

Kathy takes those very rich interviews full of the themes and histories, the longings and beliefs of the people interviewed and has them translated into English. It is from these data that she begins to build her stories. They never reflect a single interview with one respondent exactly, but in the end reflect the composite reality of those for whom the stories are created. So much so that the people are often convinced the characters are real. In effect, she is telling the people their own stories.

Her next step is to find local artists, who are often young people not yet established as artists, to illustrate the stories. These illustrations further enrich the stories, making them even more real to those who will hear them. We remember once visiting Kathy at this stage of the process and walking onto a beautiful balcony in the early morning sun and seeing maybe ten young people busy as they could be, drawing and coloring their illustrations. In some cases, they were being paid for their work for the first time in their lives.

We suddenly began to understand how every step of Kathy's work was empowering those with whom she came into contact—first the interviewers, then the artists, and finally those who would become facilitators in the classroom. At Fonkoze, we called them monitors, but they were in fact borrowers themselves. They were clients who had expressed an interest in helping to facilitate the learning of their peers. In some cases, all that distinguished them from the participants in their sessions was the fact that they could read and write.

Before you knew it, their lives too had changed. Kathy taught them a whole new way of helping others to understand themselves and their families and communities, of engaging them in a novel way of practicing new skills, of facilitating their growth, of freeing them to participate wholly in their communities. Once these monitors understood Kathy's method and had the opportunity to practice it, their lives too changed. No longer were they just small merchants struggling to put food on their tables and their children in school every day—suddenly they had become change agents in their communities, and they could recognize with real pride the impact they were having on other people's lives.

What a pleasure it was to see all the people in the Fonkoze family that Kathy had empowered even before Brigitte had enrolled in the sexual and reproductive health class! The interviewers, the translators, the illustrators, the monitors—they all reported what an incredible gift it had been to work on this project with Kathy. We could see that indeed Kathy was accomplishing exactly what Fonkoze was about: providing the people of Haiti with the tools they would need to re-create their country.

Along the way, we too became believers in Kathy's method, in her discovery that, as she articulates it, "If I tell people their own stories of romance, love, pride, happiness, humor, shame, sadness, anger, humiliation, and fear, and then engage them in a process of reflection, dialogue, conversation—this could act as a springboard for living a more just life." We have seen it bring a new light into the lives of so many people. It builds self-confidence in some, it inspires leadership in others, and it enables almost everyone to address the real-life problems they face in a fresh and sometimes dramatic way.

So years later, we asked Kathy to return to Haiti to develop a new series on children's rights. New research shows that nearly 3 percent of Haitian children are *restaveks*: child domestic workers. Families, often those in the countryside, cannot afford to feed or educate their children and so agree to give them away when promised the children will be fed and educated when they become part of someone else's family. Rarely do the benefits of good food and good education result, however. More often the children become child domestics, forced to work long hours until they are simply thrown out into the streets when they mature and perhaps become impregnated by one of the men in the family. Kathy agreed to come to Haiti and once again develop the stories that would allow learning groups to become engaged in retrospection, active dialogue, and role playing as the people practice new ways of communicating.

In this book, drawing on her years of living and working in cultures as diverse as an American Indian reservation, Ethiopia, Thailand, Bangladesh, Haiti, Uganda, and Latino and African American communities in Los Angeles, Kathy achieves what we always hoped she someday would—she opens her philosophy, her methods, and her practices to the world. For that, we are eternally grateful and hope that many others will have the privilege of learning from her.

Anne H. Hastings
Founder and Director, Fonkoze Financial Services
Director, Microfinance CEO Working Group

Steven Werlin
Faculty Member, Shimer Cllege, Chicago, IL
Regional Director, Extreme Poverty Program, Fonkoze

SEX, SHAME, AND VIOLENCE

Introduction

In this book, I refer to eight different programs of narrative practice. Each of these was developed under the auspices of various organizations (see the Acknowledgments for details). All of the projects integrated research and application in a holistic and multidimensional approach to project topics. The programs had similar goals: to change the nature and extent of conversations about program topics and to effect behavioral change. Of these eight, five are still being used and expanded in their original design and intent, two are being reconsidered for use, and one is no longer being used.

The first Haitian project and the Latino and African American projects addressed HIV prevention and sexual and reproductive health, while the Ugandan project, though topically similar, emphasized sexual, domestic, and civil violence. The second and third Haitian projects focused on children's rights and environmental problems.

The Thai and Bangladeshi projects were quasi-experimental studies. The Thai HIV and AIDS/sexual health project compared the efficacy of peer group education with health worker tutorials and written materials only. The Bangladeshi project integrated HIV prevention and sexual and reproductive health education into an ongoing health initiative and compared the impact of health promotion programs such as those involving door-to-door community-based health workers with ones involving pharmacists and clinical health educators.

Each project took approximately two years to develop from its inception to the completion of its field test and evaluation. Most projects followed a pre- and post-evaluation design, which used a quantitative survey and qualitative interviews to assess the program's impact. In all the projects, program participants met in learning groups. Ordinarily the facilitators who led the learning groups were peers of participants and were selected by the supporting organizations or by the target communities. The facilitators received training in the story topics, as well as in health and related information, and in the pedagogical methods. The training of the facilitators took approximately fourteen days to complete. (See *www.kathleencash.com* for an example of a training manual for facilitators.) After this, learning groups met in factories, schools, literacy and community centers, treatment centers, houses, and open spaces. Each learning group had between ten to twenty participants. Men and women were usually organized into separate groups because mixing men and women sometimes resulted in less honesty, more posturing and shyness, and, at times, irreconcilable arguments.

I also found youth-only groups more productive than those that mixed youth with adults. Group members who attended a program with few absences received a certificate upon completion.

Programs generally took three months to complete for any one learning group, though this depended on how often that group met per week, the length of time allotted for each session, the total number of narratives (ordinarily one narrative per session), and the amount of health or other information to be covered—the subjects, complexity, and amount of this information is related to story topics and varies by program.

All together I wrote 110 narratives for eight different projects. The narratives in each program were usually divided into five separate books with three to five stories per book along with the appropriate factual information. In this book I will use excerpts from a few stories from different programs in order to illustrate my points.

The next section offers a brief background and highlights key features of each project to serve as a reference for readers.

1. The Thai Project (1991–1995)

Demographics in brief: Thailand, a newly industrialized country with a population of fifty-three million, has an average life expectancy of seventy years.

In the early nineties, 600,000 Thais were HIV positive and 1400 per day were being newly infected (Maticka-Tyndale et al. 1994). Thais estimated that two to four million people, or 7–8 percent of Thailand's population, would be infected by the year 2000 (Brinkman 1991; Moreau 1992). HIV prevalence was highest in northern Thailand, where Chiang Mai is the largest city in the region. At that time in the North, approximately 63 percent of brothel-based sex workers, 31 percent of male patients with sexually transmitted infections (STIs), and 17–20 percent of military conscripts were HIV-positive people (Weniger et al. 1991). Northern Thai women were increasingly at risk. Between 1986 and 1991, the ratio of men to women infected changed from 17:1 to 3:1 (Pyne 1992).

Target population: The program was developed for a target population of adolescent migratory factory workers in Chiang Mai, Thailand. In the first phase of the study, the sample was 240 unmarried women between ages fourteen and twenty-four, educated to Grade 6, who had migrated to Chiang Mai to work in the export-oriented garment industry. Eighty-five of them participated in the field test of the program. In the second phase, the sample was 150 factory workers, and young men were included.

The narratives and information: The narratives focus on how culture and social expectations for young, never married women and men affect prevention. I developed three narratives: a comic book about a flying invisible condom who speaks into the ears of youth about HIV prevention; a comic book about alcohol drinking and risk to young men; and a novel about a young, female garment worker who becomes HIV positive. Health information focuses on basic knowledge about HIV and AIDS, condom use, and sexual health.

2. The Bangladeshi Project (1996–1997)

Demographics in brief: In the late nineties absolute and hardcore poverty was endemic to Bangladesh, one of the most densely populated countries in the world (with 120 million people living 2400 to the square mile). Of adults, 44 percent of women and 33 percent of men above age six had never attended school (Mitra, Al-Sabir, and Cross 1997). At that time, the AIDS epidemic was virtually nonexistent in Bangladesh—prevalence was 0.03 percent (World Health Organization 1998)—though a rural study found that 56 percent of women had reproductive tract infections (RTIs), and 23 percent of those women also had STIs (Hussain et al. 1996). Pockets of HIV infection resided in populations of sex workers, their urban clients, and drug addicts. Among commercial sex workers, one study showed that 57 percent had syphilis; 14 percent, gonorrhea; 20 percent, chlamydia; 20 percent, herpes; and 6 percent carried Human Papillomavirus (HPV) (Chowdhury, Rahman, and Moniruzzaman 1989). There were ominous signs that HIV might spread as more rural youth were migrating to Dhaka to work in factories, and because bordering communities in Nepal, India, and Burma had high rates of infection.

Target population: The program was developed for a target population of rural adults and youth. Ethnographic research was conducted with a representative sample of twenty men, twenty women, thirteen never-married boys, and eleven never-married girls, from fourteen villages. Eight focus group discussions were conducted with fifty married adults and twenty never-married adolescents. Sixty-eight BRAC health workers and 1,890 community members were trained to integrate sexual and reproductive health education and services into their ongoing work. Most participants were non- or marginally literate farmers.

The narratives and information: The narratives focus on sexual and reproductive health education; physical development; conception; pre-, extra-, and non-marital sex; expressing sexual feelings; communication about sex; safe and unsafe sex; forced marital sex; rape; STIs and HIV; RTIs; sexual dysfunction; drug and alcohol addiction; men having sex with men; domestic violence; and healthy communication. Health information focuses on human development, puberty, fertility, STIs, HIV and AIDS, condoms, contraception, overcoming impotence, and RTIs.

3. The Haitian AIDS and Sexual and Reproductive Health Project (1998–2003)

Demographics in brief: Haiti is a country with widespread poverty and inequities. The World Bank projects that the current population of eight million will reach 12.3 million by 2030 (World Bank 2014). In 1980, the gross domestic product (GDP) per capita of Haiti was 632 USD (United States dollars), but by 2003 it had fallen to 332 USD. Surviving on less than one dollar per day, 3.9 million Haitians, most in rural areas, lived in extreme poverty and had on average twice as many children as non-poor households. In 2002 the average life expectancy for men and women was fifty and fifty-four years respectively. Sixty percent of the population lived in rural areas, and 20 percent of the children in this group suffered from malnutrition; nearly half of the population had no available health care, more than four-fifths went without clean drinking water, and only 10 percent had access to electricity (World Bank 2007). At that time Haiti had a 6 percent rate of HIV prevalence and a 1:1 ratio of men and women infected between the ages of fifteen and forty-nine, the highest rates of HIV prevalence in the Caribbean region and one of the highest in the world (World Health Organization 2003).

Target population: A representative sample of approximately 160 rural adult women and men living in the Artibonite Valley participated in private, in-depth interviews and focus group discussions. Eighty-nine people (seventy-four women and fifteen men) participated in the program. Women learning-group participants were borrowers with Fonkoze, and men participants lived in the same communities as the women borrowers. The participants lived in rural Haiti, were non- or marginally literate, and worked as market women and as farmers.

The narratives and information: The narratives focus on jealousy, migration, sugar daddies, gossip, people living with AIDS, peer pressure, pregnancy and HIV, early pregnancy, men with money and women without money, infidelity, pre- and extra-marital unprotected sex, choices of youth, adults helping each other and youth, partner- and parent-to-child communication, tuberculosis, domestic violence, sexual violence, dangerous pregnancies, STIs, and partner notification. Health information covers puberty, fertility, contraception, pregnancy, HIV and AIDS, HIV testing, tuberculosis, sexual rights, STIs, RTIs, menstrual hygiene, and sexual hygiene.

4. The Los Angeles Latino Project (2002–2006)

Demographics in brief: In 2006, Hispanics comprised 15 percent of the US population, or 44.3 million people, yet they represented 18 percent of the AIDS cases. Latinas represented 13 percent of the female population but approximately

19 percent of the cases of AIDS (Centers for Disease Control and Prevention [CDC] 2008). In 2000, the proportion of women of color living in Los Angeles County diagnosed with HIV had increased from 30 to 43 percent among Latinas, while the number of white women with HIV had decreased. A startling 37 percent of women diagnosed with HIV had no identifiable risk (Mahoney-Anderson, Wohl, & Yu-Harlan 2000). Latinas have the highest risk of HIV transmission because of unprotected heterosexual sex and reluctance to discuss condom use for fear of abuse or withdrawal of financial support (CDC 2007). There was compelling evidence that men who were having sex with both men and women (MSMWs) were playing a significant role in the transmission of HIV among Latinas (Aggleton 1996, Mahoney-Anderson, Wohl, & Yu-Harlan 2000). In 2001, approximately 22 percent of the Latino transgender population was HIV positive, the highest of any group in Los Angeles (Reback et al. 2001). Their sexual partners were predominantly heterosexual married men and this, in addition to homophobia, machismo, migration, poverty, violence, and drug addiction, accounted for the high percentage of at risk Latinos living in Los Angeles.

Target population: The Latino project included men who work as day laborers and women who work as domestics, the unemployed, and transgender Latinos, most of them undocumented immigrants. The ethnographic interviews were conducted with twenty-five women, fifteen men, and twelve transgender people. The program was conducted with 103 participants (fifty-six women, forty-seven men, and fifteen transgender people). Though the average length of schooling among participants was 7.9 years, only 5 percent were literate in English and 90 percent were monolingual in Spanish. Monthly incomes ranged from 500 to 1000 USD.

The narratives and information: The narratives focus on the sexual and reproductive health vulnerabilities of undocumented Latinos living in Los Angeles, such as on drug addiction, men who have sex with men and with women, child molestation, pre- and extra-marital unprotected sex, domestic violence, youth peer pressure, transsexuality, homophobia, stigmatization, partner and parent to child communication, adults counseling and helping youth, and youth helping each other. Health information addresses puberty, fertility, pregnancy, HIV and AIDS, HIV testing, tuberculosis, sexual rights, STIs, RTIs, contraception, menstrual hygiene, and sexual hygiene.

5. The Los Angeles African American Project (2004–2006)

Demographics in brief: Though African Americans were 12 percent of the population in the United States in 2003, they accounted for half of all new HIV infections each year and half of AIDS cases. According to a 1999–2003 CDC report,

African American women showed an increase of 15 percent in AIDS diagnosis, compared to a 1 percent increase for African American men (CDC 2003). While African American women were also 12 percent of the United States female population in 2003, they represented 67 percent of all AIDS cases among all women and had twenty-three times as many newly diagnosed HIV infections compared with white women (CDC 2004, 2006). The AIDS epidemic in the black community arose from the interconnections of poverty and unemployment, single motherhood with crack cocaine addiction, incarceration of men (Wohl et al. 1998), childhood sexual abuse (Tarakeshwar et al. 2005), intimate partner violence (Lichtenstein 2004 and Cohen et al. 2000), unprotected sex with men on the down-low (men who secretly have sex with men though publicly they are in sexual relationships with women) (Denizet-Lewis 2003), concurrent sexual partnering (Fullilove et al. 1990), and sex for crack exchanges (Ratner 1993). A Justice Policy Institute Study indicated that a black man had a 32.2 percent chance of experiencing incarceration in his lifetime, and HIV infection among prisoners was four times the general population (Marushak 2002).

Target population: The target population was marginalized African Americans such as former heroin and crack addicts in day- and confined-treatment centers and in HIV positive programs. Ethnographic interviews were conducted with a representative sample of seventy people (thirty-five women and thirty-five men). Sixty-six people (fifty women and sixteen men) completed the program and received certificates.

The narratives and information: The narratives focus on men on the down-low, child molestation, prison life, crack cocaine addiction, homosexuality and homophobia, people with AIDS, domestic and sexual violence, parent-child communication, sexuality, sexual and reproductive health, RTIs, STIs including HIV and AIDS, communication between adults and youth, family support and friendship, and youth peer culture. Health information deals with puberty, fertility, pregnancy, HIV and AIDS, tuberculosis, STIs, RTIs, contraception, menstrual hygiene, and sexual hygiene.

6. The Haitian Children's Rights Project (2006–2008)

Demographics in brief: See the earlier section entitled "The Haiti AIDS and Sexual and Reproductive Health Project" for an economic overview. In Haiti, 20 percent of urban and 17 percent of rural youth fifteen years of age (mostly girls) did not reside with either parent, resulting in an estimated 650,000 children living away from their biological parents. Estimates varied, but as many as 300,000 or 10 percent of all Haitian children lived as "children living in *restavek*" (children in domestic servitude). Most children in *restavek* are between ten and fourteen years of age. It was estimated that at least 13 percent and as many as 60 percent of children living outside their natal homes were servants (Murray and Smucker 2004).

Former President Aristide of Haiti, in his book *Eyes of the Heart*, describes the *restavek* system as akin to slavery. He asserts that children as young as three or four years, predominantly girls, live in many Haitian families as unpaid domestic workers:

> Often they are from the countryside; their parents send them to the city in the hope that the family they live with will give them food and send them to school. The family that takes in the *restavek* is more often than not one rung up on the economic ladder. Most families struggle to send their own children to school let alone the *restavek*. So most often the *restavek* children are not in school; they eat what is left when the others are finished, and they are extremely vulnerable to verbal, physical and sexual abuse. (Aristide 2000:27)

Illiteracy is a major problem for Haiti. Some researchers estimate that on average 55 to 60 percent of Haitian adults are nonliterate or functionally nonliterate; most of these reside in rural Haiti. In 2001, 73.3 percent of rural children ages six to eleven attended primary school, compared with 84.8 percent of their urban counterparts (World Bank 2007).

Most Haitian parents have a fierce desire to give their children an education. Poor rural families must pay on average 5 to 6 percent of their annual income per child for school fees. To cover these expenses, many families resort to coping strategies such as selling goats, chickens, and charcoal (World Bank 2007). This, together with class stratification, the impoverishment of rural households, and a large extended family system has led to children living in servitude.

Target population: The target population was predominantly peasants—impoverished, non- to marginally literate rural Haitians. Ethnographic research interviews were privately conducted with a representative sample of 150 rural Haitians. The program was field tested with 158 members of Fonkoze's microfinance programs and with 184 participants of Beyond Borders' affiliates, such as APPLAG (The Association of Rural Community Organizers of La Gonave), the Matewan Community School network; and the Courageous Women's Group—which all support an end to children in *restavek*.

The narratives and information: The narratives focus on the physical, emotional, and sexual abuse of children in *restavek* and children in general, including punishing children; the physical, emotional, and sexual abuse of children and youth; sexual harassment; rape; child molestation; early pregnancy; domestic violence; denying children food and care; peer pressure; communication between adults and youth; bullying; overworking children; children helping children and adults helping children; and children with disabilities. The information focuses on methods for controlling anger with children; on ways of listening to, talking to, and punishing children; on how to talk to, instead of hit, children; on the points of view of children; on treating children in servitude the same as one's own children; on youth peer pressure; on different ways to care for and protect children; and on how to talk to children about health.

7. The Haitian Environmental Project (2006–2008)

Demographics in brief: See the earlier section entitled "The Haiti AIDS and Sexual and Reproductive Health Project" for an economic overview. Each year as tropical storms hit Haiti, mudslides and flooding leave hundreds of people dead and thousands homeless and affected. "The mountains have grown old. You can see their bones poking through their skins" (Smith, 2001:70). Eighty percent of Haiti is mountainous and its vast sloping, now treeless land is fertile ground for environmental catastrophes. Nearly thirty million trees planted in the 1980s in Haiti have since been cut down (without being replaced), predominantly for charcoal and wood. Seventy-one per cent of energy use in Haiti comes from charcoal. Lacking forests and tree cover, land in rural Haiti is less capable of intercepting, retaining, and transporting precipitation. Soil erosion and deforestation have become endemic, leaving 98 percent of Haiti deforested. According to UN estimates, Haiti loses thirty-six million tons of topsoil each year. Seventy-five percent of Haiti's rivers have disappeared in one generation. Potable water is not accessible to over 75 percent of rural Haitians. According to the UK Center for Ecology and Hydrology, Haiti might be the most water poor country in the world (Lewis and Coffey 1985).

Target population: Approximately 150 in depth private interviews were conducted with rural Haitian adults and youth—a representative sample of the target population. A total of 200 people completed the field test. Of these, 103 were microfinance members and 97 were participants from a collaborating non-profit organization and their affiliates (see "The Haitian Children's Rights Project (2006–2008)" section). Most participants were non- to marginally literate farmers and/or market women.

The narratives and information: The narratives focus on tree cutting; flooding; conflicts over free animal grazing; burning fields; insect pests; market cleanliness; land usage rights; negotiating with market clients; jealousy over market and agricultural productivity; controlling erosion and top soil depletion; water usage, protection, and rights; subsistence-level farming; women farmers not reaping the benefits of their labor; and mismanagement and pollution of the environment. The environmental information addresses irrigation, water conservation, the water cycle, water pollution, herbal pesticides, burning the soil, preparing the soil, and composting.

8. The Ugandan Project (2004–2012)

Demographics in brief: For over twenty years, residents of Northern Uganda had been deeply and indelibly affected by the Lord's Resistance Army (LRA) which made frequent incursions into this area, kidnapping children, killing and torturing adults and youth, maiming civilians, burning houses, stealing or killing livestock, and destroying food crops, and by the Ugandan Army who administered the internally displaced person (IDP) camps. Carol Nordstrom's definition of a *dirty* or *terror* war applies to the war in Northern Uganda, where civilians were tactical targets, where fear, humiliation, starvation, torture, murder, and community destruction became the basis for control (Finnstrom 2008; Dolan 2009). Between 2000 and 2006 the majority of people in Pader District were living in IDP camps as mandated by the Ugandan government. While people were in the camps, on average one thousand people died per week due to malaria, AIDS-related illnesses, and violence. In 2012, most residents of Northern Uganda returned to cultivating their land and gardens. While the HIV prevalence in Uganda as a whole increased from 6.4 percent in 2004 to 7.3 percent in 2011, the highest rates were in Northern Uganda at 8.3 percent. Of those infected, many were widowed during the war. Widows had the highest HIV prevalence at 31.4 percent (Uganda Ministry of Health 2011).

Target population: The target population was rural men, women, and youth living in Northern Uganda. Approximately 150 ethnographic interviews were conducted with a representative sample of women, men, and youth in Northern Uganda. A total of 650 people completed the field test in two regions of in Northern Uganda, both deeply affected by the war.

The narratives and information: The narratives focus on sexual and domestic violence, forced marital sex, rape, family support and conflict, alcohol consumption, widow inheritance, rumormongering, child defilement, impotence, digging groups (for land cultivation, gardening, and friendship primarily between women), drinking groups (for alcohol consumption and friendship primarily between men), early pregnancy, HIV prevention, pre- and extramarital unprotected sex, communication between adults and youth and between youth, parents' preference for boy children, the treatment of children, discrimination against orphans, impact of IDP camp life on youth, partner communication, cultural beliefs and practices, and sexual and reproductive health issues. Health information covered puberty, fertility, pregnancy, contraception, HIV and AIDS, HIV testing, tuberculosis, condom use, sexual rights, STIs, RTIs, menstrual hygiene, sexual hygiene, male circumcision, the prevention and reduction of domestic and sexual violence, anti-retrovirals (ARVs), and the genetic determination of the sex of a child.

The intention of community narrative practice is to transform the nature of conversations and actions and foster individual and collective capabilities. In Chapter 1, "Lessons from Others," I talk about my own early experiences in impoverished communities and how these led me to understand the importance of approaches that fostered community potential. I discuss how social research and interventions that overlook culture, emotion, and human interaction are doomed to fail. In Chapter 2, "Storytelling and Shame," I describe the significance of the two thematic foundations of narrative practice. I explain that storytelling and shame are ubiquitous to culture and to human relations and interactions, and because of this, they are central to narrative practice.

The creation and application of community narrative practice is a five-step process, which integrates research and application. The five steps of narrative practice are divided into two chapters. In Chapter 3, "The Narrative," I describe the four steps that go into the creation of narrative with examples from eight different projects. These steps are (1) conducting ethnographic research, (2) analyzing the data and designing the plot, (3) structuring the narrative, and (4) contextualizing the narrative. In discussing step 1, ethnographic research, I explain the core skills, techniques, and issues to consider when planning and conducting research, particularly in-depth, private, individual interviews. In step 2, data analysis and plot design, I describe how data from the research is converted into a composite narrative plot. I show how a plot forms as one asks certain questions of the data. In step 3, narrative structure, I focus on the public or top-story and on the concealed, under-story—how these reflect textual and dialogic transaction and how they are created in narrative. In step 4, narrative contextualization, I explain how a narrative is contextualized through character dialogue and images and how this creates cultural salience and therefore narrative credibility.

In Chapter 4, "The Pedagogy," I focus on step 5, practice. In this chapter I show how the narrative is employed in a dynamic pedagogical process. I explain how each step in this process has the intention of not only gaining participant engagement but also of creating awareness and understanding and influencing interactions. The chapter demonstrates how the process of integrating research and applying the narrative can culminate in individual and collective change.

In Chapter 5, "Evaluation," I explain different strategies I use to evaluate narrative practice. I address the ways narrative practice has influenced people and discuss how the premises of narrative practice methodologies have deeper significance beyond their immediate impact. This chapter focuses almost exclusively on some of the overriding accomplishments of and obstacles to narrative practice through the voices of people who directly or indirectly were affected by it.

Chapter 6, "An Example of Narrative Practice," is a textual and visual explication of one narrative, *Toma and Sentana*. This example is from the Haitian HIV and AIDS and sexual and reproductive health project. This is an attempt to give readers a feeling of being there through the evolution of one brief story from research to application to evaluation.

In Chapter 7, "Reflections," I conclude with observations and insights about narrative practice. I discuss these within wider concepts about the qualities of narrative and the significance of social justice, generosity, emotions, dimensions of shame, and individual and community change.

A fundamental premise of narrative practice is that education is a conversation. Education happens in everyday chance meetings when people chat at markets or in their neighborhoods. When people share stories, they are, in fact, educating each other. The experts, in any case, are people living in rural or urban impoverished communities conversing about how to meet health, social, and intimate challenges in ways that make sense to them. This book is an explication of the process of creating and applying community narrative practice. Narrative practice is an exceptional means of changing people's lives because it comes from who they are and what they hope for—from their own volition and determination to create better lives for themselves and others.

1 | Lessons from Others

When you are poor, people will never appreciate you as a person.
If they tried to know who you are that would mean that you are
somebody.

—Haitian peasant farmer, 2002

Years ago I began using cultural narratives as an educational tool. This led me to narrative practice, the subject of this book. This path was not a direct one, but one that took me on a circuitous route of trial and error. I have had many experiences living and working in different cultural settings. Each in turn gave me deeper insights into ways in which cultural narratives could effect social change.

Early on, in two very different venues, I experienced life in poor communities and saw how people's views in these communities could be reconfigured, ignored, or misunderstood. In the 1960s I experienced how culture and the material world intersected, in an American Indian Mission and in an Ethiopian village. First, I worked on a Winnebago Indian Mission in Black River Falls, Wisconsin. I grew up in a middle-class family, and though my relatives had stories of growing up poor, I had not been directly exposed to extreme poverty. On the mission I lived with Reverend Whiterabbit and his family, and over the summer, I worked with American Indian children to prepare them for their upcoming integration into local public schools. The mission had had a school for thirty-five years, and the teacher had stressed arts and crafts. Prior to their integration, the children were given a battery of tests, which diagnosed them as socially and intellectually backward. The test takers were supposed to match electrical objects, but these children had never seen most of the objects. The children lived in wooden shacks heated by pot-bellied stoves without electricity in one of the coldest areas of Wisconsin. I remember telling the sociologist who had performed the tests that it would be unlikely that any child from this mission would score well on this test because the questions did not reflect what the children knew or had been exposed to. As far as their social skills, I remember that we played many games and the children were polite, rule abiding, and lively and caring with their friends. I could see no evidence of poor social skills, though perhaps when in public school with non-Indians, the Indian children would feel shy, withdrawn, and ashamed of whom they were in the material scarcity of their world.

My second experience was in Ethiopia in 1966. I lived in a large thatched, windowless, round house with an open fire pit in the middle (there was no electricity) and a side section where cows and goats lived at night because hyenas roamed the area. I managed to get two windows built and after a time, I converted the area where cows lived (though a few goats remained) into a small kitchen with a wood stove. The dirt floor of my house was periodically washed with cow dung mixed with water, which left a hard, smooth cement-like finish. The washing removed dried cracks and unwanted insects that (if the floor was not washed regularly) laid eggs in these cracks and burrowed into your toes if you walked barefoot. As with most things, one can easily get used to living with grass-eating animals, even their bucolic emanations.

I wavered in those years from believing that we are really all the same under the surface to the opposite, that my life experiences and the material world from which I came were so different from my Ethiopian neighbors that we were viewing each other across a huge divide. I saw a child of four pick up small rocks and meticulously form them into an intricate pattern only to have an adult kick the rocks away and tell the child he was too old for that. I saw another child of five beaten for allowing a calf, which he was supposed to be herding, stray from the herd. However, I realized that a young child, by shepherding the village cows, was taking care of the family's wealth, not a task a five year old could take lightly.

I witnessed absolute poverty: the suffering of lepers with half eaten faces; the hardships of emaciated, spindly-legged women who carried huge piles of wood up steep hills; donkeys, mules, and horses hobbled in grotesque ways that made them hop like rabbits; many people half-clothed in ragged remnants of barely recognizable shirts, pants, or dresses; and children regularly leaving school without having eaten anything the entire day. Occasionally a student or a man on a market or festival day had shoes, but no one else.

One night I was awakened by a frantic child who said his sister was giving birth and would die unless she was taken to Addis Ababa. They had no money to do this. There were no clinics within four hundred kilometers, and the village midwife could not perform a cesarean. Not surprisingly, a rural woman did not want a big baby for fear of being unable to deliver it. Health practitioners who tried to get pregnant women to gain weight were unaware of this fear and attempts to fatten up pregnant women often failed (though for many there was nothing to be fattened with). I heard funerals, regular occurrences, accompanied by intense wailing. Many children died but if one could make it to age five there was a good chance of reaching adulthood. My landlady had had fifteen pregnancies and of these, three of her children had survived to become adults.

Foreigners sometimes prefaced statements with "as Ethiopia leaps into the fourteenth century," because the land system in Ethiopia at that time was feudal. Concepts born in Western policies about social equity regarding the just and impartial distribution of resources in some sense seemed irrelevant, if not ridiculous, in this context. Rather social equity related to personal, family, and community ties. Though the material world was sparse, if one ever had something, he or she would share it with friends. If I lent a sweater, later I would see my sweater walking on someone else I did not recognize. On foot, children traveled distances of up to fifteen kilometers from their homes to school and back every day. Few ate before or during school. If one had money to buy a roll, he or she would share it. To me it seemed like no one ever refused a request. There was an implicit understanding that what was mine was yours if you were a friend, or family, or from the same village.

Rural Ethiopians did not have a drive for private property (theirs was a subsistence economy) and the all-consuming attentiveness to ownership that this drive entails. I once asked two children from my village to deliver a book to an American woman living in the town. When I saw her next, she demanded that the children apologize. She accused them of stealing a banana from her house. In their minds, they had done her a favor and probably regarded her as a friend. I told her they were probably hungry (which was another likely explanation) to try to soften her. However, she was adamant, so they had to apologize, and I had to explain to them why. I could see by these children's expressions that the experience was confusing at best and shaming at worst. The only plausible explanation to the children was that this woman was from the different planet of America. Property ownership, what one viewed as "mine" and/or "yours," was complicated, and not easily resolved with an apology. The banana incident was, for me, the tip of a cultural iceberg, a small glimpse into a vast array of frozen, irreconcilable beliefs we share about each other.

When I started working in development projects, I felt these projects did not consider culture and its relevance except to ignore, disparage, or idealize it. People were identified as statistical measurements, graphs, and calculations. Culture was an abstraction, a curiosity or a political mechanism to facilitate an intervention, but not to be understood, accounted for, and seriously responded to. I never saw an intervention that incorporated the cultural values of recipients into its intent except in superficial ways.

The language of development research often consists of measuring behavior by molding it into abstractions. I saw this in the Theory of Reasoned Action (Fishbein, Middlestadt and Hitchcock 1991; Valdiserri 1989), in the Health Belief Model (Rosenstock 1974; Rosenstock, Stecher and Becker 1994; Abraham and Sheerun 2007), and in the self-efficiency approach of Albert Bandura (Bandura 1990)—all widely used to explain, develop, and evaluate HIV prevention programs. Without considering the significance of human relations and interactions, these types of theories and models assume behavior and psychological change happens due to personal mastery. Researchers' academic attraction to abstractions generated many articles about how HIV prevention should be or was working (though statistics of transmission consistently proved otherwise). I saw myriad surveys with ideological underpinnings quite in contrast to the lives of the so-called beneficiaries. Surveys asked questions, used language, and assumed values unfamiliar to respondents as in the following example, the Sexual Relationship Power Scale, used with women in marginalized communities. Here are a few questions from this scale. Each was scored on a 4-point Likert scale, where 1 is Strongly Agree; 2, Agree; 3, Disagree; and 4, Strongly Disagree.

2. If I asked my partner to use a condom, he would get angry.
5. When my partner and I are together, I'm pretty quiet.
6. My partner has more say than I do about important decisions that affect us.
9. I feel trapped or stuck in our relationship.
11. I am more committed to our relationship than my partner is.
13. My partner gets more out of our relationship than I do.
15. My partner might be having sex with someone else.
24. Having a partner at all times is important to me.
25. There are lots of good men around to have a relationship with.
27. My partner tries to understand me—I try to understand my partner.
30. No other man could love me the way my partner does.
33. I have sex with no one else but my partner.

(Pulerwitz, Gortmaker, and Dejong 2000)

The goal of this survey is to assess degree of empowerment. What is apparent in this survey is that researchers have an ideological orientation regarding interactions between women and men. Not only would it be difficult to apply the data acquired from this survey to an actual intervention, worse still, this research has a hidden agenda indifferent to respondents' lives. How will this type of questioning and analytical framework inform? The authors set up a criterion of relationship—evaluated in terms of how much or how little—assuming respondents can interpret or have ever thought of their relationships in this way. Words and phrases like "love," "committed," "more out of a relationship," "trapped in a relationship," "being quiet," "good men," "important decisions," "to understand," or being "pretty quiet" might have no meaning or might have complex cultural meanings. This instrument assumes a lot: that a man will become angry if a woman introduces a condom but not the other way; that a married woman would admit interest in other men; or that if the respondent's husband is having sex with someone else or if the respondent suspects her husband is having sex with someone else, this is related to the respondent's empowerment. The instrument assumes correlations as though there are universal ways a woman acts (regardless of culture) if she is *empowered*. What does this tool diagnose except how any respondent compares to an idealized bias outside that respondent's experiences? The authors try to replicate a model of scientific validity, but validity here is internal to the instrument itself. Beyond this, it has little.

Does research ordinarily inform application and vice versa? Traditionally, project planners conduct a needs assessment, which is a misnomer for preprogram research. Also, needs assessment is often based on the perspectives of program planners rather than on those of the recipients. Interventionists do look to research to keep informed and to write proposals. However, like two ships passing in the night, researchers and interventionists miss opportunities to jointly design projects that integrate their purposes and activities. Commonly a study ends with a few grand, bland suggestions that give little insight or information on how a project could possibly apply the results to real conditions or circumstances. Research and intervention go about their separate journeys, independent but obliquely connected to each other in words rather than deeds.

The term *intervention* assumes the urgency of an involvement in the lives of those deemed in need. Many interventions are short lived—flash-in-the-pan experiences. Many interventionists appear to be inadvertently setting up real-life renditions of "The Emperor's New Clothes." Though not the subject of this book, this fairy tale in turn has captured the understanding of the so-called beneficiaries so well that they, too, now appreciate the emperor's fineries and play along. Some interventions might have dramatic, immediate impact, but disregard possibilities for replication, expansion, and community initiative—except to hide the fact that not much is going on. Careers are made, money spent. So I asked myself, Who is better off? Do the so-called beneficiaries believe their lives are any better and do people behave any better toward each other because of this? Do they feel more hope about themselves and their communities? In many cases, I had to answer that the outsiders and the local people who run projects—who are often more comfortable with foreigners than rural people in their own country—were the ones who profited and became better off.

My first opportunity to create a cultural narrative and test out my ideas came between 1991 and 1995 when I worked in Chiang Mai, Thailand, developing an HIV prevention program for adolescent migratory factory workers. Though I was confined to certain terms of the grant, I knew from the outset that I would try out some ideas that I had been thinking about for a long time. I wanted an HIV prevention program to reflect the complexities of culture and in that context address the problems Thai youth faced in practicing safer sex.

"Thai women are virgins until they marry." I heard this after I arrived in Chiang Mai while preparing to conduct sexual behavior interviews with unmarried youth. This subtle warning from a few university colleagues suggested that my impending interviews with Thai teenagers were misguided. One Thai colleague told me, "These factory girls are good girls. It's unlikely that they're having sex." I matter-of-factly countered this with, "Even if they are virgins, don't they still need to learn about AIDS?"

I met up with the complexities of Thai virginity after conducting a written sexual behavior survey with factory girls. I wrote a pre- and post-survey—a knowledge, attitude, and perception (KAP) survey, a commonplace type of instrument often used to evaluate HIV and AIDS programs. At the end of the anonymous

KAP survey, I decided to include questions to find out whether the girls were having sex. I asked girls to check different yes or no boxes.

In retrospect maybe I wanted to disprove the admonition of Thai colleagues. My research assistants and I collected the survey and discovered that many of the girls checked the box "Yes, I have a boyfriend" or "Yes, I used to have a boyfriend." However, out of 240 girls, all of them checked "No, I have never had sex."

"I don't believe it," I told my research assistants. "There has to be at least one young woman out of 240 who is sexually active."

Up to that point, I had met the factory managers to gain permission to conduct research, but I had not visited the girls in their own milieu. A research assistant, Wantana, conducted the surveys, but she, too, had had few private conversations with the girls. One night at 10:30 pm (the girls usually ended overtime work at 11 pm), we rode out to one of the garment factories on Wantana's motorbike.

We approached the high-walled factory enclosure through a winding dark alley. An iron-grated gate demarcated the entrance. Parked outside the grounds were groups of young men, slouched over their motorbikes, patiently waiting. The night guard knew Wantana. He admitted us into the grounds, and I asked permission to walk around. The inner factory compound was completely walled and extended from the entrance gate through a wide expanse of vegetation to the concrete factory building. Outlines of trees, tables, and murky figures emerged from the shadows between two beaming neon lights that illuminated either side of the compound yard. One light highlighted the compound entrance, and the other the main door to the garment factory workroom. Girls briefly emerged one by one from the factory door and then disappeared into the darkness. Many girls had already left; some were still leaving.

As I walked around in the dim light, I began to see couples—some on chairs, others in bushes. This particular factory had both girls' and boys' dorms. A few girls were entering the boys' dorm. Others were leaving to join the young men waiting outside the wall. Ambling around, I found myself avoiding the eyes of warmly embracing couples. In one corner a young boy was singing and strumming his guitar while groups of girls and boys encircled him, carrying on flirtatious banter oblivious to my presence. I passed what I thought was an empty phone booth, but I was surprised to see a couple necking inside, unaware of the prowling stranger. They giggled when they finally saw me.

Before leaving the factory, I talked to the guard, an older man firmly in charge of the entrance gate who probably knew more about the girls' after-hour activities than anyone. The guard sat under an eave near the gate in a well-lit area. A small outdoor kitchen and his sleeping quarters bordered the guard's station. Uniformed, straight backed, and carrying a night stick, he let me know that he took his job seriously. But in truth he was not really a no-nonsense kind of guy because his rotund, cheerful, and talkative demeanor revealed his friendship with his charges. He was protective of them but running scared.

He told me, "They are all good girls. . . . They are well-behaved and polite."

So I said, "They are like young girls you knew when you were their age?"

"Oh, NO! They are nothing like girls before, when I was young. These girls have boyfriends." Perhaps he had said too much. He backtracked . . ."but they are good girls."

"Don't worry," I told him, "nothing you say to me will get back to the girls or the management here." I briefly explained our research and intended program.

As though he had been waiting for the chance to talk openly about his unruly children, the guard confessed that a few weeks ago someone wrote graffiti on the factory wall in big letters:

WORKERS IN THIS FACTORY ARE PROMISCUOUS. THIS IS AN IMPORTANT SOURCE OF AIDS. THERE IS SO MUCH AIDS HERE.

The words in Thai were aggressive—outside the norm of polite conversation. This exclamatory note referred to all the girls in the factory.

"The owner of the house next to the factory wrote these words," the guard explained. "Whoever flirts with girls here is never disappointed, but none of the girls here are selling sex. You see the boys' dorm. Some of them sleep in there with the boys. Even one night at the bus stop outside the factory, I saw a boy and girl making love. One girl was dragged out of the factory and beaten by her parents. Her friends told her parents that their daughter was sleeping with her boyfriend. I think if a girl does not allow the boy to have sex with her, the boy can't do it."

So I asked, "Things are different now than before?"

Now the guard looked at me as though I was mad. "I feel sorry for the parents of these girls. If they knew what their children were doing, they would feel so ashamed."

We thanked him and left.

In 1991 Chiang Mai was noted as the epicenter of the AIDS epidemic in Thailand, and this was an optimum time for creating a prevention program there. I believed that the complexities of HIV prevention for a Thai adolescent had less to do with competence than with consequence. The potential consequences for a girl of introducing a conversation with a boyfriend about prevention, let alone producing a condom, could be loss of respect, trust, or the potential for a relationship. Why would a young person in the midst of a romantic encounter want to risk this? HIV prevention contradicted the very essence of teen romance: being swept away. Even the thought of introducing the subject of HIV prevention to a boyfriend or girlfriend was cause for anticipated shame (Cash, Anansuchatkul and Busayawong 1995, 1999).

When I was conducting ethnographic research with young workers in their factory dormitories, I noticed that many of the girls were reading magazines. When I asked them what they were reading, they told me about the romantic stories featured in these magazines. This understanding, together with the amorous nature of adolescent Thai culture, led me to write a short novel that portrayed the complexities of HIV prevention for a Thai girl—my first attempt at writing a culture narrative.

The novelette *Lamyai* is a romance about a young woman, Lamyai, (also the name of a tree in Thailand that bears the delicious and prized lamyai fruit) who travels to Chiang Mai, works in a garment factory there, and falls in love with a young man, Tong Dee. They have unprotected sex and decide to marry. The young man joins the military and learns he is HIV positive, and, in turn, Lamyai finds out she is positive. Girl meets boy; they fall in love; tragedy strikes—a commonplace public narrative. However, metaphorically the story comes to life. The youngest daughter traditionally inherits land in Northern Thailand and is obligated to care for her parents. When Lamyai (the youngest daughter) learns she is HIV positive (at that time, leading to certain death), she tells her family she will continue to work to support them until she becomes ill. Lamyai's commitment to work fulfills the character of a good Thai daughter, obedient and dutiful to her natal family. Because I was writing about a young woman becoming infected, I had to characterize her as a *good* woman in contrast to the current Thai prejudices associated with infected women.

Lamyai is a romantic, like a typical Thai teenager. She plants a lamyai seedling when she leaves her village and tells her family, "When this tree bears fruit, I will return to you." After Lamyai dies, her ashes are strewn at the base of the lamyai tree. The life changes of the central character are compared with the maturation of the lamyai tree, and Lamyai's death, which occurs at the same time that the lamyai tree reaches fruition, symbolizes Lamyai's *rebirth*—a signification of Thai Buddhism.

In the story *Lamyai* I juxtaposed the public narrative of a *good* young woman as virginal, pure, and ignorant about sex with the critical need for young women to know and be able to talk about HIV and AIDS, condoms, and prevention. For the character Lamyai, her unwillingness and inability to talk about HIV prevention with Tong Dee had to do with a Thai cultural value that equated female modesty to goodness. This was central to the multiple social and personal risks a young woman took if she spoke about AIDS or HIV prevention with a sexual partner, particularly a casual one who she hoped would become a steady one. I realized that this paradox is at the core of young people's vulnerability, and a narrative was the best means to depict it. Without symbolically creating these counterpoints, the story would have lacked credibility. In fact, the factory girls insisted that Lamyai was a real person and asked me where she lived. They were convinced, when I said that she was fictitious, that I was hiding information to protect her identity.

Months later, after the Thai HIV and AIDS education program was completed, I decided to include the same questions in the post-survey and ask the girls whether they were having sex. By this time, we had privately interviewed many of the girls and knew which girls were sexually active. We did not know percentages, but we knew those girls who had one-night stands, those who were sleeping with a steady boyfriend, and those who were virgins waiting for an acceptable boy to introduce to her parents. At the final survey, we keyed each answer sheet so we knew the respondent. Then we provided a slotted box where the girls could drop their sheets.

The results were the same as the presurvey. To the question: *Have you ever had sex?* Everyone answered *No.* Everyone was still a virgin. Even minor wives (mistresses) answered *No* to this question. Though at first I was mystified, by this time I more fully understood the importance of a Thai girl's desire to protect her reputation. I remember a Thai study where, in a focus group discussion, one girl said that she was having sex with her boyfriend. Girls in the group were shocked, saying this girl must be crazy—not because she was having sex but because she admitted to it (Ford and Kittisuksathit 1994).

After completing the Thai program, I began a program in Bangladesh. I conducted ethnographic research, interviewing adults who said they hated romantic love because it meant that rather than being able to arrange a marriage for their children, the children were choosing their own partners. However, their children were attending school where they were falling in love against their parents' wishes, which led to more premarital pregnancies and abortions. Parents, particularly mothers, were adamantly opposed to sex education for unmarried youth particularly when it included education about condoms. Condoms for youth were frowned upon, sex education was prohibited, and there were few public discussions about sexual health except to decry immoral acts (Cash et al. 2001).

An important difference between the programs in Thailand and in Bangladesh is that in the former I was working with adolescents living outside their home communities, and in the latter I was working with youth and adults within the rural community where they lived. Early on I appreciated the significance of this. Three Bangladeshi doctors, in full support of a greater contextual understanding of vulnerability, began conducting interviews along with me about sex and sexuality in one rural community. In one of our first interviews, a young Bangladeshi boy told us, "My father beat me for giving a girl a mango." The boy said that he loved this girl and planned to marry her, but his father would not accept this. Another discussion with three teenage girl cousins was revealing. They lived in the same extended family household. Two girls were silent as the oldest girl spoke:

I feel a thrill inside of me. I feel love with a boy. He is the neighbor of my friend. I saw him there. At the beginning I didn't notice him. He asked about me to his friends and informed them that he is in love with me. Since then, that boy wants to talk to me and if we meet on the road, he calls me to come closer to him. But I do not go closer to him to talk. One day I went to my friend's house and we talked. Gradually, I became weak. Until now, the boy does not know I am weak to him and inside my mind I am in love with him. Yet I maintain distance from him.

The next day we arrived at the same village but our reception was cool. A leader told us that we were not welcome saying, "You cannot continue your interviews here. The father of the boy [who gave a girl a mango] complained." After this, we were shuffled back and forth between a rural hospital and a development office—neither wanted us to conduct interviews on their turf. Each organization might have been risking its reputation. We eventually settled on conducting the interviews at a local microfinance office—a place removed from home, village, and the eyes of the community.

One impact of sexual diseases is that people cannot talk about them because they expose that which should have remained hidden. Feeling shame about desires and acts makes having a conversation about those things a difficult challenge indeed. When program planners and practitioners think about ways of preventing the transmission of HIV, violence, or, for that matter, any of the other countless ways people harm each other, they have failed to pay attention to what is most essential, ambiguous, and consequential about humans: their emotions. Didier Fassin's comments about health policies could apply as well to health programs: "They are not fleshy enough, imprisoning their analyses in systems of norms and institutional problems. They do not allow us to see the men and women in charge, their beliefs and interests, what they disagree about and fight over" (2007:35).

I believe emotions, especially feelings of shame, seriously challenge possibilities for the reduction and prevention of vulnerability. The condom is a good example of this. Because of its connection to sex and sexual disease, the condom entered a vast cauldron of misunderstanding, misinformation, and miseducation. Early in the AIDS epidemic, Dooley Worth wrote a seminal article about condom use (1989). If health educators had paid more attention to Worth's examples and discussion of why vulnerable women will have problems with condom use and had incorporated these ideas into their programs, HIV prevention might have had more chance of success with women at risk.

In over two thousand sexual and reproductive health interviews I have conducted with Haitians, Latinos, African Americans, Bangladeshi, Thais, Ugandans, Nigerians, and Malawians, I have heard only a handful of times that a married woman wanted her husband to use a condom. Yet countless brochures and articles contain fabricated stories of a woman trying to get her spouse to use a condom though he refuses. These pamphlets suggest how a woman should ask her husband seductively and nonthreateningly. Health advocates equated condom use in a marital relationship with empowerment. To whom were the creators of these materials listening? Some advocates of this belief invoked the words of HIV-positive women, who, after being infected by a husband, unequivocally stated that the husband refused condom use. Who can refute this: the now-dead husband? Perhaps these women were blamed for their husband's infection (a common occurrence), and they wanted the interviewer to think well of them.

"Use condoms," the most common HIV prevention mantra, assumes that transmission is the consequence of an act by an individual, similar to the drug prevention mantra, "Just say no to drugs." I found that the potential relational loss caused by introducing a condom into an intimate relationship exceeded the perceived risk of acquiring a sexually transmitted disease. The condom not only challenged sexual pleasure but also what people wanted others to believe about them (Cash, Anansuchatkul, and Busayawong 1999).

In every community where I have worked, I heard public narratives that increased risk and private suffering. These cultural narratives heightened vulnerability to such an extent that I believed it would be unlikely people's lives would improve unless these narratives changed. For one thing, public narratives often purposefully hide the underbelly of private suffering. Invariably this underbelly sets up a contradiction between the public and the private. Though we all have contradictions in our lives, for marginalized, impoverished people these paradoxes have dangerous, at times life-threatening, implications. The question for me was how could I create stories that could transform those public narratives that were inflicting, sustaining, and increasing vulnerabilities?

People fear being shamed by their social group in resource-poor communities. There, people's dependencies on one another are fragile. One cannot ever move too far from the watchful eyes of one's neighbors. Distributing what one has acquired is expected, and while this diminishes the gains of any one individual, giving back cements family and community affiliations. Jeopardizing these relationships could lead to social suicide. In impoverished communities, fear of shame and possible ostracism boosts the strength of public narratives and their effect on people's actions.

A vulnerable, often poor person can hardly confront an oppressive person, social group, or situation. Too much is at stake. Shame-filled paradoxes cause timidity and silence. On the other hand, in Thailand I saw that when the factory youth were given certificates stating they were sexual health advocates, they spoke about HIV prevention with their partners, their families, and their communities. They told me that this symbol of credibility gave them social protection and inhibited questions about how they, as young people, knew about HIV prevention. From this, I realized it was possible to give people the tools to speak in ways that lessened fear of reprisal.

In impoverished communities in the developing world, there are few material resources. Face-to-face communication is the norm; there is virtually no technology to interfere. Not surprisingly, people in poor communities suffer less from anonymity and loneliness than people in the industrialized world, though in the intensity of constant everyday contact, there is the possibility for abuse as much as assistance. Nonetheless, I think that the potential for collective change within poor communities is their greatest resource.

Finally, I learned that one commonality of humans is the proverbial elephant in the room. Focusing on colorless, cultureless, emotionless language and imagery—outside the realm of *real* human experience—means not speaking to the shameful in everyone's sight. Most communities have many elephants, and these are as ubiquitous to culture as human efforts to ignore or hide them. "Sites of disempowerment are not just simple matters of human rights issues emerging from women's economic and sexual servitude. Rather, romance, hope, pleasure, need, . . . and abuse are interconnected sites through which agency is asserted and (dis)empowerment experienced" (Yea 2005:457).

I felt if I could tell people their own stories of romance, love, pride, happiness, humor, shame, sadness, anger, humiliation, and fear, and then engage people in a process of dialogue, it could act as a springboard for living a more just life.

2 | Storytelling and Shame

Storytelling

I have rarely been any place where I am not greeted, enthralled, and entertained by a story. In the late 1960s, I was living in a remote Ethiopian village. The evening ritual there is to go to someone's house in a neighboring compound to talk and drink coffee. In the round houses, a thick center pole emerges out of a dirt floor and rises up to an intricately woven thatch work of bamboo beams. Smoke from a cooking fire encircles the beams, leaving a deep black-brown residue and the distinctive smell of charred bamboo and eucalyptus. A blackened coffee pot balances on three stones in the middle of the center fire. Everyone sits on small stools encircling the center fire for the primordial practice of storytelling.

A story begins as the coffee percolates. The mother of the house and an older daughter serve the circle coffee and hard, shelled, roasted grains. When one old man speaks, he captures everyone's attention. He is called the wizard. His plots and deliveries excite the senses. The silence of the listeners is only broken by expressions of group affirmations such as "yea" and "aha" and sometimes laughter or small private exchanges that break off—short interludes until the wizard resumes.

I remember a lively conversation in which a student explained gravity. It started when I tried to describe where I came from and how I got to Ethiopia. One neighbor asked me how I managed to travel without falling off the earth. Another neighbor asked me if Haile Selassie was the king of my country. Everyone was puzzled by the student's explanation of gravity except the wizard, who asked questions until he understood. Then, following a hands-on demonstration in which the student used an orange as a prop for the earth, the wizard launched into a story about a boy who leaves his village and travels the earth without falling off of it. A good storyteller is a sense-maker.

What causes our obsessive attraction to television other than the endlessness of a storied world? Perhaps the residual damage of television is not to the story itself but in the loss of artful storytelling as a practice of engagement. We as TV viewers are bereft of the storyteller, of his or her performance, guidance, and availability to nurture questions and conversations. Lacking direct contact with a face and its voice, television seduces us onto a minefield, stripped of reflection. There is lag time. The poignancy of a moment is gone when the reaction is delayed or never cultivated. On news programs, within seconds of hearing about the deaths of thousands from bombs or an earthquake, we are throttled with an ad about the best way to wax a table. In the practice of storytelling, whatever wizardry the storyteller can conjure up, switching from human catastrophe to a shining table is not likely. It is a point of logic as well as morality: the more distanced we are, whether by culture or by miles, from a storied event, the more immune and unresponsive we are to its lasting consequences.

From childhood, stories teach us how to be good, moral, and just. Stories teach us how to solve problems, how to meet crises. They give us models of heroes who overcome obstacles that we ourselves might someday encounter. By hearing a story about the "other," we learn about the self. Stories are the essence of our entertainment. Stories scare us, flatter us, and vicariously take us to places we will never see to encounter people we will never meet. Yet we think we know them because we know a story about them.

The social function of stories is global—universal to the self and to our social interactions. In the well-told story, we hear, feel, and see that which is most essential to us. Communities flourish when people demonstrate care for each other. After hearing the story of a family problem or crisis, people are drawn to help the needy. A story can also bind people to the rules, and to the consequences if those rules are broken. A story can stigmatize. What do young women fear more than a sexual story about them that will forever label them as easy? The harness of culture is told to rapt listeners with a subliminal admonition: This might happen to you if you do this. What better way to enforce obligation and moral injunction than by a repeated story about those who transgress? "Narrative or storytelling is the most ubiquitous and powerful discourse form in culture and in human communication" (Bruner 1990:77).

Culture, as Clifford Geertz points out, is always local, always particular, however universal its aspirations, fulfilling an inner point of view as one interprets the world in concert with others. The world "in concert with others" is the shared symbolic world of human culture, "an ordered system of meaning and symbols" by which humans define, interpret, and give meaning to their world (1973:50). Causal explanations of human experience (such as that unprotected multiple partnering increases the risk of HIV transmission) cannot make plausible sense without being interpreted in light of this shared world of meaning. Culture mediates dialectical tension between social reality and individual existence, between knowledge and experience (Berger and Luckmann 1966). Nowhere is this more evident than in the shared stories people tell about themselves to like-minded others, stories that mediate and are mediated by human experience.

What does storytelling or narrative do? Narrative discourse is essential in bringing experience to conscious awareness, meaning, and memory (Ochs and Capps 1996). We have no other way to describe lived time than in the form of narrative discourse. It is inseparable from life. Narrative discourse becomes the power to renegotiate the meaning of the past and construct future meanings (Mattingly and Garro 2000). As Walter Benjamin observed, "Information needs immediate verification. Nothing lasts beyond its immediate use, but a story does not need explanation. A story expends itself over time" (1968:89).

Narrative discourse is also about the situated self or how one is situated with respect to others and to the world (Bruner 1986). The storyteller creates meaning by which the self can regulate, reaffirm, and transform its relations with others. Hannah Arendt described the deep-seated strength of storytelling: "Compared with the reality which comes from being seen and heard, even the greatest forces of intimate life—the passions of the heart, the thoughts of the mind, the delights of the senses—lead an uncertain, shadowy kind of existence unless and until they are transformed, reprivatized and de-individualized, as it were, into a shape to fit them for public appearance" (1958:50).

Stories about Sex and Power

Few things in the world inspire us, create hope and shame, consume our loftiest and basest emotions, imprison and liberate us, titillate everyday conversation, and create uproarious laughter more than our stories about sex. As a child, I heard stories about my relatives, one who spent a good deal of her married life having sex with men other than her husband, and another who occasionally appeared at his own door in earrings and a dress. As a child, I could never tell whether these people were envied or pitied, but I knew that their escapades entertained and captured everyone's imagination at otherwise mundane family get-togethers.

We are also imprisoned by such stories. We had a suspected pedophile in our extended family. Or let's say an older male who sometimes acted inappropriately with girl children. This was not talked about in public conversations, but only behind closed doors where the abhorrence of his behavior was magnified by secrecy and doubt. These were private conversations that prompted protective behavior. When girls in the family were small, mothers were careful to never leave them alone in a room with this man. As these girls grew to adulthood, those same mother-protectors made sure those daughters knew.

Families often protect the pedophile or wife beater or sexual misanthrope against outsiders who might expose that family member and thus the weakness of the entire clan. "Don't wash your laundry in public" is axiomatic.

Emotional paradox is particularly unique to sexual storytelling. Sexual storytelling transforms the relationship between the private and the public and creates agency in the face of disempowering circumstance (Jackson 2002). "Power is everywhere in sexual stories" (Plummer, 1995:28). Sexual storytelling can achieve legitimacy when stories of private pain shift into the public domain. This way, shared secrets become publicly interpreted and meaningful (Wa Mungai and Samper 2006).

Women's stories of sexual violence exemplify power and powerlessness in the text as well as in the telling, in the interactions between the teller and the audience and among the audience. Storytelling about sexual violence sets the common-place against ruptures in human behavior. Private plight achieves a public persona within dynamics of resistance and suffering, love and betrayal, desire and abandonment. What binds the audience is not only the particulars of suffering, but also the emotional resonance and recognition of ever-present power: "What makes power hold good, what makes it accepted, is simply the fact that it doesn't weigh on us as a force that says no, but that it traverses and produces things, it induces pleasure, forms knowledge, produces discourse. It needs to be considered as a productive network which runs through the whole social body, much more than as a negative instance whose function is repression" (Foucault 1980:119).

People live in complex interactions with others. Sexuality, as Simone de Beauvoir observed, is a lived experience, as is culture; all are commonly held lived experiences that produce and reproduce themselves in everyday interactions.

What's Shame Got to Do with It?

In 1995, after I had been in Haiti a few weeks, someone comes to my door asking me to visit a woman dying of AIDS. I follow this person through tangled, dusty undergrowth to a deserted hut set far away from others. The hut has a dirt floor in the middle of which is lying an emaciated woman, naked except for a filthy sheet mottled with bodily excretions half-covering her body. Streams of unfiltered sunlight encircle her. After I enter, the room quickly dims as curious faces crowd the two unscreened windows. At the dying woman's side sits a woman with a nursing baby. The woman's job is to clean diarrhea away from the sick woman's anus with a piece of cardboard. There is no source of water in the hut except for a small cup with a few tablespoons. There is neither soap nor anything that can be used to clean the diarrhea-covered dying woman or the piece of cardboard being used to clean her. The woman with the nursing baby tells us that her baby has diarrhea. Barely audible, the woman with AIDS whispers to me, "What's wrong with me? Am I dying?" As we are leaving, the woman's uncle, who owns the hut, says that his niece slept with many men. He blames her for the shame she brought to his household. She dies the next day.

Some months after these events, the director of the hospital where I was working told me that an influential donor had informed him that ethnographic research and educational programs are not useful and what the hospital needs to do is identify which people are HIV-infected and let their communities know. I thought, "If you do this, it is one grotesque way of ending the misery of people with AIDS. People will ostracize them and they will die." The hospital funds a home care program and discovered early on that it is not reasonable to inform the community of a person's HIV status. Home care participants fear that anyone, including members of their immediate families, will find out. Confidentiality is promised. On one occasion I witnessed frantic parents follow the visiting hospital staff to their vehicle, asking why their daughter was so sick. Sometimes the staff delivered medicine to clients far from their homes. With this strategy, questions from family or neighbors were muffled, as was the hospital staff's fear of inquiry.

Haitians (and others) have told me that HIV counselors should not tell an HIV-infected person his or her status. In their opinion, pronouncements like these sever the infected person from his or her family and community, breaching social and sexual bonds and thus hastening death—not from the virus but from shame. Many times I heard comments like, "Do you want to be humiliated?" or "You will humiliate your family!" directed at someone who was putting him- or herself at risk for HIV. I also heard—simply put—"Who would want to have sex with someone if they knew that person was infected?" At a time when HIV infection was certain death, is this sentiment difficult to understand? Didier Fassin gives us a moving account in the words of a person living with AIDS, of his aloneness and anticipated shame: "Sometimes when you need a person it's hard to say, 'Hey, I'm just like this,' because you must have heard that most of the people, when they hear you are HIV-positive or you have AIDS, they won't agree maybe to stay with you or to make friends with you. It's the most difficult thing that a person can ever experience" (2007:207).

Shame and, inversely, pride, are ubiquitous emotions, preeminent in our emotional-relational lives (Darwin 1872; Nietzsche 1886; H. Lewis 1971). Our daily interactions are constantly being tested by an immediate experience of or an anticipation of shame (Goffman 1959). Shame, because it is a social emotion (Scheff 2003), not only results from what one is, but also how one looks to others (Williams 1993; Wollheim 1999; Morgan 2008).

Shame, why it is felt and how it is expressed, is intrinsic to culture, to who and what we are. In Thailand I frequently heard the phrase "loss of face," a common reference to shame and a metaphor for the utter disappearance of public identity. Relentlessly connected to our social fears, shame lives because, as Cooley wrote, "We live in the minds of 'others' without knowing it" (2006:208).

Shame is a vital thread, woven into the human psyche, strengthening and fracturing social-sexual bonds. Shame is not subversive. Shame just is—an all-enduring reminder if not a presentiment (Probyn 2005). Shame and its truculent offspring, humiliation and rage, are in response to feeling "Who am I that I am wronged? Why am I being wronged?" or "Am I being wronged because of this wrongness within me?" (Wollheim 1999). We feel shame at the experience or threat of failure. Not able to discard or ignore it, shame can evoke beauty as well as ugliness, catapulting us into collective maniacal revenge or to altruistic acts of generosity. Shame is a constraint within ourselves that we cannot separate from—"an unalterable presence of I to itself" (Levinas 2003:64). Levinas describes the commonplace metaphoric nakedness of shame: "What shame discovers is the being who uncovers himself" (2003:65).

Shame is commonly reflected in religious rituals, texts, and symbols. In two archetypes of Western religion, there is hope in shame's revelation and atonement—the nakedness of Adam and Eve in the Garden of Eden and the near nakedness of Jesus in the crucifixion are proverbial metaphors for the utterly exposed self before ultimate power. In religious ceremonies, I look through the liturgical texts for references to shame. Many are oblique, but this one is direct: "O my God, in You I trust, Do not let me be ashamed; Do not let my enemies exult over me. Indeed, no one who hopes in you will ever be put to shame" (Psalms 25:2–3). According to this passage, trust in God will free one from the inescapable. I realized after living with American born-again Christians in Uganda that their trust in God supersedes all else. HIV-positive Ugandans willingly convert to born-again Christianity. Freedom from shame is both practical and redemptive.

Shame fosters objectifications. One can become a bad girl, a secondhand wife, a weak husband, a dangerous AIDS carrier. Stigmatization exposes fragile mirrors, telling us things about ourselves we do not want others to know. Because it is socially conceived, shame is contagious. Stigmatization extends to the family or friends of a stigmatized person. In the case of a never-married girl, labeling her as sexually loose extends beyond her character to the characters of those who befriend her. Once she is identified as easy, it is likely that a boyfriend or husband will not be able to trust her. Is it not likely she will also be loose with others? What does this mean about a man's value if he is willing to marry or cohabit with a woman of dubious worth? Stigmatization can become a spiraling demise, especially for the marginalized—the poor, homeless, formerly imprisoned, or emotionally ill.

Our social existence is forever being negotiated, and when negotiation fails, as it often does, we experience emotional paradox between our inner desires and our social expectations, between what we want to believe about ourselves and how others see us or respond to us. At the same time, we long for coherence. We want to set it right. What does that mean, to set it right?

In Malawi I witnessed how a public performance against shame affirmed community solidarity. When the hidden text becomes unmistakably, unambiguously visible, contradictions need to be resolved. I attended a ceremony where an unmarried girl was being prepared for marriage. The cultural obligation of the old women present was to tell the girl the secrets of marriage. The primary secret to be revealed in a secluded hut was a reenactment of childbirth. Unfortunately the girl had already given birth. The old women were angry. They began the ceremony by chastising the girl in public about her pre-marital pregnancy. The women surrounded the girl who was lying on a blanket and yelled at her. She cried. The secrets of childbirths were going to be told, but not before everyone acknowledged that this girl had committed a breach. The old women realigned the predicament of this paradox by taking back what was denied them. How can they teach her the secrets of childbirth when she has already given birth? As keepers of the ritual, the old women embarrassed the girl and thereby reasserted their control. In this case, shaming had a ritually healing function—not for the weeping young girl but for the public good. For the moment, the paradox was resolved.

However, what if the right becomes the ruthless? Whether grounded in ethnicity, race, nationality, religion, or personal feelings, when shame provokes, it often demands compensation. On a grand scale, consider the Holocaust or, more recently, Bosnia, Rwanda, and Darfur. Consider the election of Ronald Reagan in the wake of America's loss of the Vietnam War, or America's assault on Iraq after 9/11. Can public discourse redefine shame before humans seek revenge or unleash some cumulative mad desire to identify who is responsible and attempt to close the paradox forever? I leave this historical question to others. What I am suggesting is that the experience of lived contradiction can create a seething, excruciating effluence that is not easily resolved. So leaders emerge to manipulate whole societies into blaming others by subverting shared-shame into perverse acts of collective retribution.

Anthony Giddens believes that in social-sexual bonds within the modern world, shame is repressed but ever-present (1991). In America, for example, repressed shame is license for relentless publicly televised sexual discourse and hyperbolic expressions of desire. In turning reality into a spectacle, television is a gaze castrated of its power to shame (Miller 2006). Perhaps, as Scheff and Retzinger believe, the modern world denies shame as a defense against the loss of human bonds so beleaguered by the pervasive myth of individualism (1991).

One distinction between human bonds in postmodern America compared to non-industrialized societies is that in the former, one is expected, and in the latter, one is obligated. Obligation implies there are social requirements outside individual proclivities. In rural Haiti, for example, a common expression is "I am obligated." When a man and a woman marry, they are not just obligated to each other. Intimacy is contingent on bonds external to the couple. People do not always fulfill obligations, but social sentiments believe they should. In developing countries, one is obligated to family and local community first. This does not mean that people do not have choice (as outsiders often interpret), but it means that the family domain, rather than an impersonal one, circumscribes one's field of choice.

Most cultures outside of the industrialized world are societies of *we* rather than *I*. This might explain how conceptually the self appears to have different significances in these contexts. In industrialized societies, people see themselves as individuals, each having a unique identity, whereas in developing societies one is a person, which has greater social than individual significance (Taylor 1985).

In small communities, particularly those that are resource-poor, conservative, or highly stratified, social stigmatization can lead to social death. Private texts are concealed from public expression. Following this reasoning, an AIDS sufferer, if socially exposed, could cast severe aspersions on him or herself and his or her family. No one wants this. In rural communities, keeping the lid on is a fundamental requirement for social harmony. Sometimes we are mystified by how a seemingly peaceful community can suddenly erupt. We cannot fathom what spark ignited this eruption, because we do not understand accumulated hidden tensions. When something becomes part of the public conversation, we should not assume that people did not know it already. When someone openly casts doubt, if not slander, underlying social fragilities are exposed to public scrutiny. Small communities are ill equipped for the emergence of the shameful anomaly. Reaction to a person or a group who causes undue public shame is to blame, reject, stigmatize, silence, isolate, desert, cast out, and in rare cases, stone and kill. Most societies have some history with this.

Sex and sexuality, in particular, undress us to the possibility of failure through unacceptable, forbidden, and unmet desires. A person's hidden shameful desires or acts can easily be blamed on a group, if not on the individual who openly expresses what the condemner would have liked to remain hidden. For such an accuser he would have preferred "let sleeping shame 'lie.'" How unfortunate that the birth pangs of the AIDS epidemic were first heard through the halls of supposed unmitigated sin: homosexuality. In many quarters, heterosexuality is principally valued for its reproductive potential. In industrialized societies, women have achieved separation between reproduction and sex. When sex is disaggregated from reproduction and sex becomes the 'property' of the individual (Giddens 1992:27), public acceptance of sexual diversity is possible. Modern women, no longer exclusively valued for fertility and its associated family obligations, changed the sexual landscape of industrialized societies. Where heterosexuality is concomitant with procreation (endorsed by religion and state) and when one's sexuality is the property of family and community, homosexuality can hardly be tolerated as an alternative male enterprise. As a result, in much of sub-Saharan Africa there is outright denial that homosexuality exists within one's own people. Some countries in this region have concocted the belief that homosexuality is something outsiders introduced. When the self is utterly out of reach, blame is leveled at aliens or the insidious infiltration of interlopers, a proverbial roadblock to anticipated shame.

Shame and Reciprocity

In Marcel Mauss' seminal work *The Gift* (1990), he interprets sexual relations within the notion of reciprocal exchange. The legitimization of a socially and sexually recognized exchange is symbolically affirmed in marriage. In customary marriage, a woman and man, because of the gift, are obligated to each other. After an initial exchange, once a bond is socially established, must the gift be repeated for this bond to be sustained? Marital or steady bonds extend far beyond the coupling pair usually legitimized through social recognition rather than by repeated regular exchange.

As an example, in Uganda bride price is the gift of cows, money, household goods, and/or alcohol in exchange for the bride in order to solidify family relations, to show appreciation to the girl's family, and to instill community recognition of the marriage. One can mistake this exchange as the commoditization of women. All else follows from this perception of women's subjugation: domestic violence, forced sex, transmission of sexual diseases, and so on. I do not believe this is an apt interpretation of gendered exchanges. Bride price might involve hours of fluctuating negotiations where alliances are made, shifted, and remade. Some are public and others hidden, creating and forming relationships and attachments far outside a gift's strictly reproductive meanings. By ignoring the intricacies of emotion within the exchange, we lose sight of the deeper influences in social and intimate interactions. We see the performance of culture, its cognitive display, rather than its affective underbelly.

The inherent fragility of the intimate heterosexual bond is embodied in the many ways that rituals and practices brace it against dissolution. This bond ensures the continuation of family, tribe, ethnic group, and culture. When continuance is threatened, intimate bonds can dissolve. In this next example, a Ugandan woman has given birth only to girls. In Uganda a daughter or woman cannot inherit property and therefore a family needs a son. When a man who does not have a son says, "Where will I rest my head when I die?" or "Who will bury me?" this man is asserting that without a son, without familial transference of land, he will lose his ancestry and thus his identity. Here a Ugandan woman articulates her and her husband's feelings of shame because she has failed to give birth to a boy:

> My husband said, 'My cattle are producing, but you are not producing. I am tired of feeding your anus.' He keeps money for drinking. I have six daughters. I can't divorce because my brothers have used my dowry. [If she divorced, her natal family would have to return bride price to her husband's family.] I was the only daughter in my family. When he gets angry he says to me, 'You are producing only prostitutes. No one will remain to bury me.' Sometimes he refuses to buy food to cook and medicine for the children. I feel useless. I feel so much shame.

Wherein does this woman's shame lie? The dialectical encounter of this woman's objectified social loss is set against her personal feelings. This woman desires social approval and acceptance; however, she has failed to comply with a fundamental obligation of the marital/social contract. What she desires cannot be achieved, and her identity as a good wife and mother is in question. Would she be better off in another place where producing a male child is not tied to her social identity? Or are cultural values so internalized that anywhere she ventures, she would feel she is a failed woman? I believe this woman's identity is tied to her social significance. If she was no longer subjected to the shaming gaze of others, her feelings of loss would in some ways diminish.

Ugandan men talk about how they feel shame when their wives ask them for things they cannot provide. Poverty intensifies feelings of embarrassment and humiliation—emotions arising from shame. A man explains: "Poverty contributes to a lot of abuse. I am not able to meet my wife's demands like buying meat and salt. I feel ashamed. During times of poverty, I become too rude. Then she does not make demands on me."

At the same time, women in Uganda and many other places shame their husbands because they believe he is giving away what is rightly theirs: "Having a partner outside marriage is normal to me if the man can fully support the woman at home. But what hurts me is the fact that this man is failing to support his existing family and now puts on another burden."

In Haiti as elsewhere I heard similar comments: "When he has money in his pocket, he doesn't know you. He gives it to other women. I fight with him about this. When I ask him for money, he doesn't give it to me. He gets very mad. But when he needs something from me, then he gives me money."

When reciprocity fails, power often surfaces to set things right or to close the paradox (as mentioned earlier on a larger scale). This next example of a Bangladeshi woman's explication of forced marital sex is fraught with ambiguity. Her shame is rationalized with explanations that her husband's satisfaction will bring peace or that she can do nothing to stop it. However, she is resisting sex because her husband has failed to fulfill his obligations. There is no reason to believe that this woman has low self-esteem. She experiences a paradox where her subjective self is set against the depersonalization inherent to acts of extreme violence—in this case, sexual violence. This is a shame-filled discovery:

> We cannot refuse sex. The result will be unhappiness, because whenever the husband feels it is necessary, he applies force. He might not care for the children . . . does not give food or clothes or care for the home. If the husband can be satisfied there will be peace. Sometimes I give false information saying I am sick or menstruating. When he tries to apply force then I tell him to go away. Women cannot refuse. Almost all husbands apply force. When my husband is strong, he copulates three or four times in a night. I feel sick. Force is bad for health and mind. If we do not have fish and rice, how can we have sex?

Publicly, ideology trumps personal desire, but privately, it is often the other way. Because the gift of reciprocal exchange that established a marital bond in the first place is not sustained over time, this absence of exchange can become the under-story of marital shame. Shameful contradictions lead to anger and subsequently to violence and a host of other problems that dramatically increase vulnerability. Nothing has prepared men and women to live harmoniously nor is that necessarily the social intent. Not surprisingly, shame is mitigated by social or family alliances as much as it is caused by them, as a Latino woman explains: "He wanted to have sex with me. I didn't. He became aggressive and started to hit me. I knew he was going with other women. I couldn't say anything because he was so aggressive and I was scared. He forced me to have sex. I didn't think about leaving him because I didn't want to look like a loser in front of my family."

The Uses of Shame and Narrative

Shame can arise from an absence of human solidarity—what one as an individual has collectively failed to do (Levi 1959, 1989). Levi metaphorically describes the utter collapse of human solidarity in his poem "Monday," saying that no sadness can compare with a lone train, "That leaves when it's supposed to, / That has only one voice," except a cart horse chained to a life of isolation, "Shut between two shafts / And unable even to look sideways" (Levi 1988:11).

The intentional destruction of solidarity among prisoners in World War II concentration camps led to unmitigated shame among survivors. When Jewish survivors of camps requested they be buried at the site of a former camp (Langer 1997), were they asserting a solidarity in death that was denied them in life? Was knowledge of this possibility a means of alleviating shame?

Solidarity within the gay rights movement overturned sexual shame and public narratives about homosexuality. The proclamation of gay rights in the United States and in other industrialized countries probably did more to stem the tide of HIV than any collectively inspired disease prevention effort in human history. When gay people came forward and publicly claimed their sexual identity, their communities were attempting to banish shame and fear. As gay rights coalesced with safer sex, gay people asserted a critical means of reducing their risks. They opened up, laid claim to and expanded public conversations about being gay. They broke with a historical, stigmatized silence and combined it with the how-to of HIV prevention. Nevertheless, in conservative communities, a gay person who publicly expressed his or her identity would have risked social suicide or worse. Then, too, the rights movement for many gay people was initiated outside the communities in which they grew up. Many, in order to confront shame, had to remove themselves from their natal communities.

There is a profound silence surrounding things about which people feel shame. In economically poor communities respondents tell me they fear other people will ridicule them if they know about their intimate problems. During interviews, they repeatedly say, "This is an issue in my bedroom. I told nobody about it." Respondents fear public exposure, such as this man who asserts, "One day I beat my wife because she followed me up to where I am socializing with my friends. She did this because she had been hearing from her women friends that I had an outside love. I don't want people to know about sexual issues between my wife and I. This will create shame between us."

A woman, for example, might appeal to her partner for money for food by highlighting his inadequacies. Her partner, in his inability to fulfill his obligations, feels shame and in turn shames her. Each will inflict shame because it has been inflicted. Shame is retaliated in patterned responses as people live and relive emotional and relational paradox. While social patterns are observable, patterns of intimate interactions are less observable.

Repetitive feelings of shame turn into silences or damaging discourses or outright acts of violence, furthering an inability to speak. How are injustices and inequities structured into human interaction to perpetuate contradiction? Can these contradictions be redefined? How can we overcome the pervasiveness of harmful shamed silences? In essence, how can we reconfigure shame?

Stories are vital to therapy. Dream interpretation, for instance, is the weaving of seemingly illusory events into a sense-making story. Storytelling is vital to the therapeutic process of healing, significant to the meaning of individual and social suffering (Mattingly 1998). "Voice is the most precious of human endowments" (Kleinman 1988:29). Suffering normally deprives one of voice and, therefore, the hope that others might respond is lost. Reclaiming voice and reconstituting the self is a critical therapeutic process (Frank 1995; Sharf and Vanderford 2003).

However, the therapeutic process that engages a client in narrative discourse assumes that there is something wrong with the individual. Feelings of shame are attributed to low self-esteem or personal pathology caused by that wrongness (or vice versa). In an educational process where the social world is publicly questioned, though, the wrongness of the person is not. Enhanced self-confidence results when community dialogue reinterprets shame-filled subjectivities. "Shame can be useful—by warning us that we are subject to an external criticism that we have accepted and internalized and that we should consider seriously the justification and the truth of that criticism" (Morgan 2008:42).

When I began thinking about the possibilities of creating a reflection of shame in a cultural narrative, I asked myself if a narrative could be merged with pedagogy and whether this process could achieve a dialogical practice. I wanted to create a cultural construction of reality within a narrative structure that mirrored shame. I wanted to show how characters spoke and got into emotional and relational conundrums similar to the audience's. In essence, I wanted to be able to tell people their own stories and use these as a springboard for conversation.

The purpose of narrative practice is to influence the way people talk about and respond to shame by influencing awareness, private and public conversation, and thoughts of the self in relation to others—in essence how we talk, what we say to others, and subsequently how we act. This praxis of shame can create a democratic response because it levels the playing field of private suffering and demands a reconfiguration of it. This reconfiguration of shame is a response of *I*—I must hide my vulnerability from others—to a response of *we*—how our private plights are shared. In sharing private plight, we can reflectively renegotiate past hidden texts of suffering and transform shame. So I asked myself: How can sentiments of shame become an impetus for constructive public discourse? How can the context of social, cultural, and gendered vulnerabilities be used to inspire individual and collective change? How can individual acts of courage, of leaving one's private hiding place and showing who one is, in disclosing and exposing one's self (Arendt 1958:186), lead to acts of generosity and justice? To answer these, I created a transformative community narrative practice.

3 | The Narrative

Step 1: Ethnographic Research

In Northern Uganda I learned that forced marital sex is a common source of humiliation and intense conflict between husbands and wives, often precipitated by alcohol. I wrote a story about forced marital sex, leaving ideas about reconciling, coping with, or solving this problem up to participants. In some parts of Uganda, kneeling to greet one's husband is a sign of respect, as is providing bath water and food when he returns home. When there is marital discord due to a husband's failures, a wife often refuses to do these things. After the program, women explained that forced marital sex was no longer a problem. One group laughingly told me that for Christmas, their husbands bought them cloth—a sure sign of love. The men said that their wives now respect them: "I would demand food and a bath from my wife because she didn't respect me. Now she welcomes me and takes my bike and brings me bathing water without me asking her. I feel this program has instilled discipline and respect for me. My wife now values me. The neighbors can confirm this. Sex is based upon the consent of both." Some women said, "There is love between my husband and me now." However, when I see a woman genuflecting before a man, I blanch—a touch of shame. This is not an image that would fare well in my culture. But when participants tell me there is more peace and happiness in their households, who am I to assume otherwise? Ways of reaching an amicable equity—not clear-cut or non-ambiguous—have cultural resonance to which I have no real experience, authority, or obligation. I do not have to face the everyday challenges that others must face. We must be conscious of our assumptions and how these might color our interpretations.

Changing Assumptions, Changing Responses

I conduct ethnographic interviews to gather descriptions and interpretations of events that can be used to create composite stories. I try to capture actual dialogue that a respondent (the person being interviewed) uses in recounting an event. I am looking for interpretations that uncover the feelings of *self* within the event, as well as the feelings of *the other*. During the interviews I am learning how human relationships evolve, dissolve, or reconcile as I unearth, through respondents' emotive recall, culturally relevant descriptions of people's vulnerabilities.

Central to the interview process is determining what questions to ask and how, when, and where to ask them. When training interviewers, I use the example of this question: "Does your grandmother's ghost ever bother you?" This might be a question a respondent would ask if he or she was the interviewer, but one that would not have occurred to an interviewer coming from a Western perspective. This encourages interviewers to learn the respondents' beliefs, which will help them formulate meaningful questions.

Much has been written about different types of questioning and therefore I will not belabor this point. It is worth mentioning that open-ended questions beginning with phrases like "tell me how," "tell me something about," "can you explain that more fully," or "what happened then," are critical to ethnographic research. However, a first question that requires a *yes* or *no* or a factual answer is a useful way to begin talking about a sensitive subject. This first question can ground the respondent. For example, the interviewer might ask as a first question, "How old were you when you had your first sexual experience?" or "Have you ever been in love?" Subsequent questions might begin with "Tell me something about. . . ." Beginning a conversation about a sensitive subject with an open-ended question might be too unnerving, too forward for most respondents.

When I started training others to conduct ethnographic research, I developed a question guide that would not limit the skills of a researcher or the spontaneity of a respondent. I needed a guide so the data from the different interviews and interviewers would have some semblance of consistency. For my own interviews, I informally jotted down question categories. However, for research assistants I created a general topic, an overall objective for the topic, and two categories of questions, primary and secondary. In this chapter I will focus on interviews about sex, sexuality, and sexual behavior, but the ideas in this chapter could apply to a broad range of interview topics.

A common problem for beginning researchers is that they ask two or more questions simultaneously without waiting for a response. Because there are few guideposts, the interviewer might be anxious, particularly if the respondent takes a long time to answer. Or, following this reasoning, the interviewer will ask a few questions as though searching out loud for a question that will work. Most likely, because the respondent does not understand the question, he or she cannot answer it. Most non- or marginally literate respondents ordinarily will not directly tell an interviewer that they do not understand the question. Differences in their statuses do not allow for this. The interviewer should ask one question and try to clarify it before pursuing others.

Sexual initiation, for example, is often an introductory topic in a sexual behavior interview. The primary question might be, Can you tell me about your first sexual experience? Secondary questions, asked one at a time, might include: What happened? How did you feel? How do you think the other person felt? What happened in your relation with that person? Were you afraid? If so, of what were you afraid and why? Did you tell anyone? If so, who? Why did you tell that person? What happened in your relationship with that person who you told?

Each question ultimately limits, directs, obscures, or expands the respondent's interpretations. One question can redirect an interview and reveal a completely different interpretation of an event. Here is an example:

I was in rural Haiti with a beautiful, robust young woman who was HIV positive, as was her baby. Her husband, an older man, gaunt and tired looking, was not infected. He had been living in a city, and his young wife, with their two children, had been living in a rural area. I took a young Haitian doctor with me for this interview. The doctor was popular with his patients because he has the ability to put them quickly at ease. I told the doctor, "We are going to ask this young woman questions to find out how she interprets what has happened to her." The focus of the interview was on the economic reasons she chose to engage in unprotected sex with someone other than her husband.

She painted a picture of her extreme poverty. She told us that her husband, who was working as a tailor in the city, was not earning enough to support her and their two children. She explained, "This man [the one who infected her] bought food and clothes for us." She wanted to make it clear to us that she had had few boyfriends in her life. By telling us that she did not start sex until her early twenties and that she had had only two partners in her life, she is telling us who she is.

Her characterization of the circumstances that led to being infected was classically drawn—she did it because of poverty. Then I told the Haitian doctor that we were going to change the focus of the interview. I asked him to ask her about the man who infected her: "What was he like? What was sex like with him? Did you love him?"

The young woman was embarrassed. She laughed and told me that she couldn't discuss this in front of this man. I promised her the interview was confidential and reiterated that this man is a doctor and he respects the personal stories of his patients. The young woman then launched into a description of how beautiful the man who infected her was, how he was built, how he looked, and how sex with him was exciting. She sheepishly grinned, broadly smiled, and laughed with pleasure when she thought back to her relationship with him. She told us she was in love with him. Clearly, her decisions were not devoid of sexual desire. But she also needed money. Often it is difficult to separate these things: physical and emotional attraction, attachment, and security. When we asked this woman about condom use with this man who infected her, the woman giggled, "Yes, at first he used a condom. But then he stopped using them." I asked why. "Because I asked him to."

After leaving this young woman, we discussed how changing a question can completely change what a respondent will reveal. It was not only poverty that motivated this woman's sexual decisions but also emotion and desire. By characterizing women as only victims of poverty we overlook their humanness and their potential for agency.

Changing a question changes the understanding of events that, in this case, led up to the woman's infection. What was interesting about this woman is that in the beginning of the interview, prior to questions about the man who infected her, she spent much of the time talking about how she only had sex with her husband and the man who infected her, telling us that she started sex late in life and that she had been brought up as a good girl, unlike other girls in her community. Whether this was true or not is immaterial. What is important for the interviewer is to make note of what a respondent wants the interviewer to know about him- or herself. These small things are noteworthy because they reveal information about what the respondent and her or his community value. The woman's husband was not infected. This was deeply stigmatizing for his wife; so she wanted us to know she was a good woman.

Reducing Noise

When I first started conducting sexual ethnographic interviews, I noticed that my most successful interviews were more like conversations than a structured interview format would allow. Once respondents relaxed and no longer felt like they were being interviewed, conversation flowed. Sometimes I turned off the tape recorder. From then on, the person began revealing things that I had been struggling to find out when the tape recorder was on. By visibly turning off a tape recorder, I was removing an outside interference.

The tape recorder is an example of what I call *noise*, not because of sounds it makes but because of its presence. In preparing for an interview, I look for possibilities of reducing noise, those things on your person and in the environment that might color what the respondent tells you. Noise can be almost anything: your clothing, your shoes, the way you walk or talk, how you seat yourself, the place you choose for the interview, or the equipment you use.

Noise cannot be avoided, but it can be reduced. Anything that is invasive or unfamiliar to the respondent's senses will create noise. My presence, regardless of the environment, is already causing noise. I am an outsider asking insiders about sex. What could be noisier than this? My appearance and everything about me is foreign. I can only guess what the respondent is thinking: "Why did she choose me? Who is this woman asking me about sex? Why does she want to know about me in this way?"

Gender and age differences can create noise. If the interviewer is a man asking intimate sexual questions to a female respondent, most likely the response will be dishonest or superficial. In most venues, women do not reveal private information to men outside their immediate family. Besides this, a husband might take great offense at a strange man asking his wife intimate questions. While it is less problematic for a female researcher to ask a man intimate questions, his response might also be unreliable, but for different reasons. Men add sexual bravado to their responses if a female interviewer is young or perceived as sexually available. In some venues, it might be assumed a female interviewer is propositioning a male respondent. I remember standing in a park asking a handsome young man if he would agree to an interview. He pointed to a young research assistant and said, "Yeah. I want her to interview me."

I am older than most of the people I interview. Gray hair, for a sexual behavior researcher, is an advantage. In many venues I represent a non-sexual being. Out of respect, a young interviewer cannot ask the questions I ask as an older person. When I interview youth, my age causes feelings of security for some and embarrassment for others. For one thing it is a rare adult, in their experiences, who asks questions as sexually explicit as mine. For some, the interview becomes a source of comfort in being able to talk about things they had never talked about before.

Words can cause noise, because they can cause alarm. Once I use a highly charged word, I see a change in the respondent's attitude toward the interview. I avoid the use of the word AIDS or anything connected with it. The mention of AIDS evokes a cauldron of premonitions, judgments, and, for some, shame. At the end of the interview I might ask about the respondent's understanding of HIV and AIDS.

Using a word like *restavek*, for some people a pejorative term for a child in servitude, might force the respondent into defensive posturing or into a political camp. Referring to a child in servitude as a *slave* can also open up a host of emotional reactions. Because many of the interviewer's questions could contain provocative terminology, the interviewer needs to learn what the problematic words are and avoid using them, while the translator needs to know how better words can replace offensive ones.

One way to reduce noise is to establish from the beginning why you are talking to the person and what you want to talk about. Evasiveness casts a cloud of suspicion. After introductions, I give a brief, clear explanation of the purpose for the interview (saying something about its relevance to a future health program), the need for the respondent to be honest, and the promise of confidentiality, and then I get a verbal or written agreement from the respondent for the interview. After a brief chat with the respondent about herself or himself (to help her or him relax) and about myself, I might ask this question: "Can you tell me about your first sexual experience?" This question immediately grounds the respondent and allows the respondent to choose what he or she wants to talk about.

Choice is significant. When you think back to your first sexual experience, assuming you have had one, think about your memory of the event, what you might choose to tell an outsider, and what you might selectively eliminate. However fragmented a respondent's selection of events, it is critical to the interview that this first question and subsequent initial questions create an open field of response. A good interviewer will use this open field as a starting point for other questions. Later, during data analysis, patterns and meanings will emerge from uninterrupted descriptions punctuated by well-placed, probing questions.

Translating

To create a composite narrative when I am working outside English-speaking communities, there is a four-step process. It begins with the local-language interviews and progresses to the translation of the interviews into English, then to writing the narrative in English, and finally translating the written narrative back into the local language. In each language change I am concerned about losing important data. Frankly, the ability to create authentic narrative dialogue rests on the skills of translators.

I work with translators to make sure that a research question is not being translated directly to respondents because it must be revised so that it makes sense to a respondent in his or her own language. Bilingualism is not the only competency good translators should have; they must also understand the nuances, slang, and subtext in a respondent's use of language. These are related to social class, ethnic group, locale, wealth, education, and age. I, in turn, must generally know these in order to select a competent translator.

Translation is challenging because translators who are versed in their own language and in English might want to paraphrase or summarize. When I initially began conducting interviews, it was comical when a respondent spoke for a few minutes, sometimes becoming quite emotional, and then the translator delivered the respondent's words in affectless seconds. For example, a respondent might say, "My wife said terrible things to me. . . . She threw my belongings out of the house and locked the door. She shamed me in front of my neighbors." Translator: "He says he fights with his wife."

When I first started interviewing people, a translator accompanied me and translated during the actual interview. This interrupted communication and having this odd language (English) interjected into our conversation caused discomfort for the respondent. When I trained others to conduct interviews, they used tape recorders and later translated those recordings into English. In Uganda, I was told that respondents would react negatively to the use of tape recorders, largely because of Uganda's recent political history. Instead of using tape recorders, I trained interviewers and note takers together. The note taker wrote the translation simultaneously in English as the interview was being conducted.

I found this kind of simultaneous translation effective because I could immediately read the translations and work with the translators and note takers to improve their skills. When there was a long delay between the time of the interview and the time I received the translation, it was more difficult to retrieve missing information.

I asked the note takers to record the interviews in the first person as though they, themselves, were the respondents. Having a respondent's words translated in the first person helped me create narratives. As I read the interviews, I felt I was in the presence of and closer to the respondent's inner world. This kind of translation also enhanced the skills of the note takers as they became more responsive to the subjective interpretations of respondents.

Listening

Finding Coherence

When a person talks about personal experiences there is coherence, though she or he is not necessarily conscious of it. When I listen to a good interview, I hear coherence. Effective, well-placed questions inspire valuable respondent interpretation. Sometimes when respondents interpret their sexual selves, they are in essence recreating themselves as they go along. Out of fragments comes a kind of coherence. However, these are not the usual trappings of a story. If the interviewer asks a respondent to tell a sexual story about herself or himself, sometimes the respondent is stymied; the story is a forced, reconstructed recollection; or the respondent selects a public story about someone else and makes it his or her own. Some respondents are more comfortable talking about other people or things heard on the radio or from public media. When the interviewer asks for a sexual story, what is told is aberrant—something titillating, heard from an anonymous source.

Men, in particular, often want to present themselves as upstanding and moral. Their stories are at times more like platitudes of how others should live than real insights about themselves.

Conflicting feelings that occur because of a sexual experience are patterned over time into the repeated story. Usually the practiced story is not revealing because the intent is to hide something. These are *umbrella stories*, honed, weathered exhortations and repetitions, insulating the respondent. There is comfort in them, but for my purposes, they are similar to what one hears in a focus group discussion—stories that support public beliefs and norms.

Listening for Red Flags

I tell research assistants to listen for red flags as the interview-conversation proceeds. Red flags are verbal alerts, things being said or implied by the respondent that seem to be causing or increasing her or his discomfort. With research assistants, we brainstorm possible sources of and reasons for red flags.

A red flag is a signal to the interviewer to probe more deeply into a respondent's recollections and interpretations. Obvious red flags are oblique references to child molestation, physical and family violence, unwanted sexual initiation, and drug addiction, and these are often accompanied by emotional expressions of humiliation. An interviewer's skill at being alert to these red flags improves as she or he becomes more familiar with the interviewing process.

To probe, the interviewer must learn a critical skill: attentive listening without judgment. This leads to questioning guided by the conversation or, as I call it, interviewing on your feet. The skill of active listening needs practice. The interviewer attunes herself or himself to the language, conversation content, gestures, facial expressions, and other bodily cues that reveal things related to but possibly outside of what the respondent is saying. Most importantly, it requires that the interviewer ask a next question based on the direction the respondent is choosing at that moment. Only through attentive listening can the interviewer facilitate this direction. If questions are preplanned, the respondent's voice can be lost in the interviewer's goal of fulfilling the objectives of the instrument.

Talking about sexual experience can appear evasive, contradictory, and complicated. Sometimes a respondent conceals something that the interviewer thinks important or wants to know. I tell assistants, "When you are interviewing don't give the respondent the feeling that you are sex police. Then you've created an interrogation, rather than an interview." Some interviews are rich and insightful; others short-lived and sparse. Some respondents are loquacious and seemingly honest; others talkative and insincere.

Listening for Patterns in Truth and Lies

Is veracity important? Lying, like truth, is patterned and revealing. In Bangladesh I found this to be true when I asked men about domestic violence. In one interview, a man asserted how well he treated his wife and espoused female equality. He asked me to take a photo. When his wife stood up to join him in the photo, he pushed her behind him. Maybe he wanted the photographic image to reflect her subservience. Or perhaps others would have judged him harshly with the impropriety of a photographic image of his wife on the same footing as he was. All I knew was that in that push, there was contradiction.

Feelings of shame relating to sexual betrayal sometimes define people's recollections. A seminal event, like being molested at a young age, is sometimes believed to set a pattern for all subsequent sexual experiences. One male respondent told me, "The fact that I was molested when I was seven by a thirty-year-old woman affected all my sexual relationships after that." Whether his experience of child abuse really determined all his later sexual choices is irrelevant. What is relevant is what a respondent believes.

Respondents hide things. However, a suspected lie reveals as much as an overexposed truth—sometimes they are even one and the same. In one interview, a respondent told me repeatedly that as a married man he had only one sexual partner. He refused conversation, pushing the interview into a short-answer format. At the end he asked me, "Is true that a man can get rid of AIDS by having sex with a young woman?" He had requested the interview with me. I believe he hurried the interview so he could get to this question.

Another time I interviewed a woman who was being physically abused by her husband. A counselor recommended her. She was difficult to interview. Respondents who have been abused in the past talk more openly—there is less reason to hide anything. A formerly closed text can be opened because it is distant. But a raw text, an open wound, is fragile. If the respondent is being abused at the time of the interview, he or she might resist personal disclosure.

The interviews are not intended as therapy, though some respondents have said that the interview helped them unburden themselves, and because of this they felt better afterwards. I do not press people to talk about what they are resistant to reveal, if I believe this will harm the respondent.

Listening for Actual Dialogue

I ask respondents to tell me what was said during an event or conflict. Respondents say things like, "I kept asking him if he has a woman outside." However, to create dialogue in the stories, I need more detail. I repeatedly ask what was said between the respondent and his or her partner. The emotional intensity of the event is a basis for recall. Often and understandably, shameful words are attributed to the other rather than the respondent. Since I want to create real conversations in the narratives, I cannot rely on interviews with a gender-biased perspective. In order to create dialogue between story characters, I must get both perspectives about what happened and what was said. For example, when a man's wife reports that he married a co-wife and there is conflict between the husband and the first wife, I need to find out what she said and what he said. I can then get a full picture of what dialogue occurred between them. Knowing culturally significant words, phrases, and dialogue is essential to creating a credible story.

Focusing on Events

I find that when questions elicit feelings, they arouse memory. For example, a respondent might begin by describing how her husband took another partner. She describes events that led up to this. If the interviewer asks, "How did you feel?" at a point where one might expect intense emotion, this frees up a cascade of descriptions. Self-absorption, a focus on *I felt* or on a vivid explanation of feelings is common in conversation in highly industrialized countries. When a respondent is non-literate, more likely from a developing country, I find that asking about feelings does not lead to an elaboration of feelings but to a deeper description of events. Non- or marginally literate people are unused to psychologizing conversations. Generally I format questions to begin with a question about an event and then later on ask a question like "How did you feel?" regarding a particular event. This also allows the respondent to comfortably expand. The respondent will then describe the event in more detail adding his or her emotional response but within a fuller, deeper description of the event.

Feelings are embedded in events. However, if the interviewer focuses on events without reference to emotions, descriptive data will be externalized from personal experience. The data then will sound cold and dispassionate.

Here is an example:

Interviewer: Can you tell me about your first sexual experience?

Respondent: He was the first person I loved. We worked together. He was good looking. He dressed well, and he knew my parents. I talked to my friends to see if he was good.

Interviewer: What did they say?

Respondent: They said I should take my chances. But that's what they always say.

Interviewer: Can you tell me about your life together?

Respondent: We were together four years and then we got married. He didn't have any other people at that time. We got used to each other. We didn't have any big conflicts. Finally, he had other women. He would give them what I worked hard to get.

Interviewer: How did you feel about that?

Respondent: I realized he didn't want me. He didn't really love me. He told me that I didn't have the right to ask anything from him. He had so many women and other children.

Interviewer: How did you know?

Respondent: They made gestures to let you know they were with him. He wouldn't listen to me. I knew he was bad for me. I just stayed by myself and worked to raise my two children.

Interviewer: What happened after that?

Respondent: He went away for eleven years. And then, after all that time, he came back.

Interviewer: What did he say?

Respondent: He didn't say anything. He came back into the house carrying all his clothes and hung them on the wall. He just settled back in. What could I do? It was his house. I couldn't put him out.

Interviewer: What did it feel like for you after he came back?

Respondent: He would try to talk to me. Touch me and tell me that I am his wife. But I just ignored him. When I made food, I would give him a little—coffee, bread, banana. I would wash his clothes because if I didn't, then people would speak badly about me. I was obligated to do it. But I had really closed my heart off to him.

Interviewer: What did you say to him?

Respondent: I said, "See, you never imagined that you would turn into an old man with no money and then, the women would not want you anymore."

Interviewer: What would he say?

Respondent: He would ignore it or say, "Oh, let's not talk about that. C'mon, you are my wife."

Interviewer: How are things now for you and him?

Respondent: Now he doesn't have other women because he doesn't have any money. We have six years since we have been back together. We don't really talk. We just live our lives and do what we need to do. It is his house that we are in.

Choosing Time and Place

An interview must feel friendly and unhurried. Ordinarily, one interview can last from one to three hours. I like to choose places that are private, comfortable, and away from family and friends. In villages, it is difficult to find privacy. In homes I arrange a time, if possible, when a respondent is alone. Sometimes a crying baby interrupts, and the interview stops with a promise of return. Sometimes children run in from play, and their mother must respond. Not surprisingly, children want to hang around out of curiosity and see what this outsider is asking their mother. Generally, if an interview is interrupted or stopped early on, the interview will not be satisfactory because the spontaneity that might have occurred in an uninterrupted interview will not be achieved. When this happens, I reschedule the interview. Sometimes it is better to start over.

In rural, small communities where neighbors see and report on unusual activities, fellow researchers and I sometimes drew unwanted attention. As mentioned previously, in rural Bangladesh, two Bangladeshi doctors and I ventured into a village and conducted a short interview with a teenage boy. When we arrived in that village the next day to continue interviewing, the village leader asked us to conduct our interviews elsewhere. To conduct uninterrupted interviews, it is often better to choose a neutral place, outside the respondents' milieu, with a margin of safety and with a degree of familiarity.

Being Aware of Limitations

There are limitations to any interview. Besides limited time, the respondent might have limited reflexivity to deeper layers of experience. However meaningful the interviewer might believe an event, a respondent may not have thought deeply about something that took place many years ago. By trying to peel away layers of experience, the interviewer would be acting as a therapist. The interview is not intended as therapy, though the interview might end up being therapeutic as I previously mentioned.

An interviewer can spend hours on any one significant event; however, an interviewer should look for conscious, easily accessible interpretations of experience. If the interviewer ends up psychologically probing the respondent, the construction of recalled events can become too detailed, overly subjective, marginal, or even outside normative interpretation. The respondent might make up information on the spot. The respondent cannot necessarily remember or does not really know what to say to overly detailed questions, but in an effort to please the interviewer, the respondent will come up with information that the interviewer appears to want.

Instructing and Practicing

I have worked with over 150 research assistants. Some did not require much instruction. Others found thinking on their feet challenging. Some interviewers want specific questions rather than categories of information and general questions. Some of them imposed assumptions about sex and sexuality on others from their own experiences. The interviewer must be cognizant of his or her personal assumptions so that questions do not subvert the interview into what the interviewer expects or wants to hear.

One would think that being of a similar culture to respondents would be an advantage. Not necessarily. At times I found university students difficult to work with. Not only was social class an obstacle, but also they had been trained in survey research methods. They had limited capacity to listen, to suspend judgment, and to even take off their urban trappings to interview rural or less educated people. Some were difficult to retrain. How much formal schooling one has does not necessarily correlate with interviewing capabilities. For a rural, not formally educated Ugandan woman, failure to receive adequate bride price might be shameful, while for a university-educated, urban Ugandan with a degree in gender studies, it might be the opposite—a testament to liberation. During the Latino program, one researcher had a master's degree in women's and Latin American studies and spoke convincingly about her love for the poor, but at a staff meeting, this researcher told malicious jokes about the obesity of poor Latinas. Individuals who genuinely like people and enjoy relaxed, convivial conversations without prejudice toward respondents, without reactive ideological biases, have been my most adept researchers. Of course, good analytical skills are essential as well.

To train researchers to conduct this kind of research, they must practice and be given the chance to improve in the skills of listening, engaging people in a directed conversation, and knowing how to focus on what the respondent is saying in order to probe. Usually I work with researchers over a four to six month period at each venue. During that period, we meet regularly to share and discuss our interviews. I use these meetings as opportunities to train and review data. Interviewers also critique their colleagues' interviews and sometimes have suggestions for better ways to ask questions than my guide advises. Such meetings build rapport and support between the researchers. I can also directly see whether the primary and secondary questions are retrieving the kind of data I want. Because I do not feel bound to the initial interview guide, I adapt questions or add questions when necessary.

I ask researchers to be aware of the reactions and emotions of respondents if these add significance to what a respondent is saying. Nonverbal cues such as a respondent's overall emotional state, posture, and so on can contribute to my understanding of the data. I ask researchers to take note of these.

During the training of researchers, I involve them in one hands-on experience before they begin the actual research. A practical hands-on experience is necessary because unexpected difficulties arise (like with tape recorders or note takers) that need to be sorted out before the actual fieldwork begins.

There can also be problems with *noise*. In the morning of one practicum in Haiti, interviewers met over breakfast. Some were wearing noticeable jewelry, and a few women were wearing short skirts. Because they were interviewing people in a rural area, I asked them to take off their jewelry and to change into long skirts since this was appropriate dress in that locality. One interviewer objected to this imposition. After a day of interviewing, they returned and one of the young women who had changed to a long skirt recounted that she had interviewed a born-again Christian teenager and that if she, as the interviewer, had been wearing a short skirt, the respondent would not have opened up to her.

I require that researchers conduct ethnographic research ethically. Before each interview, the respondent must agree that he or she understands that the interview is voluntary and confidential. For non-literate respondents, a statement that describes confidentiality must be sensitively crafted because concepts of *voluntary* and *confidential* are new and might cause suspicion (though a sexual behavior interview in itself is also, for most, new). Additionally, I encourage interviewers to talk to the respondent in ways that are respectful, friendly, and honest. Most respondents will readily speak openly when they feel that the interviewer is genuinely interested in them and willing to listen.

Furthermore the interviewer must be straightforward, cautious, and aware. During an interview the respondent might see the interview as a source of future assistance where there is none. Thus the interviewer must be careful not to mislead the respondent into having this belief.

One critical aspect of interviewing is difficult to teach. I try to describe this aspect by telling a story about myself as an ostensibly failing interviewer. I was in Croatia interviewing a Bosnian refugee who began to tell me stories of horrific cruelty she had witnessed. I believed at that time that a good interviewer must remain neutral and objective. However midway into the interview my eyes started tearing up, and I involuntarily started weeping—tears flowed from my face onto my notes. I apologized and told her I wanted to stop the interview until I recovered. I knew this was not acceptable behavior for a good interviewer. When the respondent tried to comfort me, I felt even more embarrassed, as though we had switched roles. She told me she appreciated my emotional response, which was unlike other interviewers who had not reacted to her stories. Later she invited me to her apartment and prepared food for me. Thus, in indirect ways I continued the interview and learned about the lives of Bosnian refugees in ways I would not have if this incident had not occurred.

I speak with interviewers about seeing within a respondent a reflection of oneself, as in the mantra "There, but for the grace of God, go I," not out of pity, but out of the belief that this person in front of me could be me. I am not suggesting that the interviewer do what I did or fake emotional connection, but an interviewer must recognize commonalities within the respondent, if not in experience at least in sentiment. My best interviewers have been those who identify with or are from similar communities as the respondents or who authentically care about and want to learn from them.

Over many years I have conducted and facilitated over one thousand ethnographic interviews in very different settings. The purpose is to learn about sex and sexual experience; or for the Ugandan project, about domestic, sexual, and civil violence; or for the Haitian children's rights program, about the treatment of children; and for the Haitian environment program, about environmental problems. I generally conduct individual interviews because, while group interviews are informative, people tend to say what is publicly acceptable rather than individually revealing. One acquires richer, more meaningful data from private, individual interviews. From among the individual interviews, one can draw comparisons to get a sense of what is not being stated publicly.

In the process of collecting and analyzing ethnographic data, patterns emerge. These patterns will inform the creation of a composite narrative. Any one narrative must reflect a recognizable verisimilitude in people's relations and interactions. In a sense the composite narrative is similar to a public narrative; however, as the reader will see, this narrative also contains an under-story or a story that defies a commonplace public narrative. In the next three steps I will describe how a composite narrative is created and formed.

Step 2: Analyzing Data and Designing the Plot

I was walking with a girl who has an uncanny ability to find an iguana in a tree or a salamander in dead leaves. No one understands how she does it. As we walked in a forest, she suddenly stopped. "There!" she exclaimed. She pointed to tangled bushes and whispered, "Snake!" At first I was skeptical. I didn't see anything but motionless green matter. Then she gave me the exact location by putting her hands on either side of my head and gently moving it like it was a telescope looking for a celestial speck. All the while she was whispering directions. And then I saw it.

I said, "How beautiful! Amazing! How do you do it?"

"Patterns," she said. "You see patterns, but you look for disruptions. When you see one, your eyes grab it!"

As an observer of humans, I, too, see patterns. Whether we focus on a snake languidly sleeping on a branch or on a respondent describing a shameful encounter, we begin with patterns. Then I pay special attention to disruptions because these are the seeds for narrative.

Looking for Recurrences and Patterns

Sometimes I have more than a thousand pages of interviews and notes in front of me. I read over the data many times. I look for patterns and themes and recurrences in events, in language, and in dialogue. Reading one interview, I can see patterns in what any one respondent talks about and in how he or she speaks, but I am most interested in patterns across interviews.

Once I have a good overview of the content, I start highlighting repetitive responses. I pay attention to patterns in statements, phrases, conversations, and expletives. Then I extract the repetitions from the data and start sorting them into separate categories such as what women say, what men say, and what youth say. I keep each of these categories on separate sheets, and I move data around or add new categories when necessary. As I analyze the data, I create more categories with greater specificity, such as what women say about domestic violence, early sexual initiation, or forced marital sex; or communication about sexual health from the point of view of parents and of children; or what a husband and a wife might say to each other in a specific crisis such as when a malicious rumor has discredited either one.

I pay attention to exceptions. Respondents might tell a story, sometimes outlandish. The story, while interesting, is not reflective of a common story; it is an anomaly. Other people repeat these stories and one could easily be drawn into their cultural significance, but they are stories to shock—not an experience of the many but of the few. On the other hand, the story about child molestation in the African American program (which is described in Chapter 3, step 3) might appear to be an exception. However, the target group was crack cocaine addicts, both men and women, who exchanged sex for drugs. Many had experienced childhood abuse. The narratives must reflect experiences of the people for whom the project is created.

I ask researchers to note the reactions and emotions of respondents if these give significance to what the respondents were saying. I take note of these divergences in the interviews because these can contribute to my understanding of the data.

As I analyze data, I also think about how the narrative plot will relate to the pedagogical process, how the plot might be interpreted in practice. At the same time that I am paying particular attention to the structure, language, and images in a story, I am also thinking about how the story will provoke testimonials, questions, role-plays, and dialogue.

Asking Essential Questions

In a narrative plot, I try to create a realistic, composite interpretation of the complexities of power and powerlessness. However, the composite narrative is not an ideal representation of how life should be or a characterization of good versus or over evil. In order to do this, I ask seven essential questions when analyzing data and forming the plot:

- What are recurring problems in the data that speak to serious sexual and reproductive health (or children's rights, or environmental issues, depending on the program)?
- How do public narratives interpret these problems?

- Who are the central characters and how will their relations and interactions heighten or reduce the problem?
- What cultural events, encounters, beliefs, and practices might directly or indirectly contribute to vulnerability?
- What is the logic of shame and silence in this narrative production of vulnerability?
- In what ways might this narrative project possibilities for change in conversations and actions?
- What activities in the pedagogic process—discussion questions, role-plays, and medical information—might inform and transform the public narrative?

A realistic story must reflect the ambiguities of human interactions. For example, if a sexual partner in a story suggests condom use, the person suggesting this might be risking a shameful encounter. So I must portray the interaction of the two subjects in the context of what that suggestion might mean to the subject (who is suggesting use) and to the object (the one who it is being suggested to), taking into account the gender of said subjects.

Shame emerges within human negotiation, within the evident potential for loss or gain. Within the harnesses of culture, people try to prevent, reduce, confront, aggravate, or escape the possibilities of shame. In this regard, any topic or problem within the composite stories must reflect the ways people try to accomplish these.

Though the contexts were decidedly different, research data from eight different sites revealed similar causes of vulnerability such as sexual and domestic violence, poverty, unsafe sex with multiple partners, poor communication between and among adults and youth about sexual and reproductive health, personal histories (i.e., crack addiction), or cultural beliefs and practices (i.e., a preference for boy children or violence between neighbors over land). Here I will use one story from the Ugandan program, *Widow Inheritance*, to show how a composite story plot was formed in answer to these questions:

What are recurring problems in the data that speak to
serious sexual and reproductive health (or children's rights,
or environmental issues, depending on the program)?

The Ugandan program story, *Widow Inheritance*, focuses on the problems of a family when one brother dies and one of the deceased man's brothers is obligated to marry the widow. Before I began interviewing, I was aware of this practice, but I was told that because of the AIDS epidemic, no one inherited widows anymore. However, while I was interviewing and analyzing the research data, I learned otherwise. Entire families had been infected as one brother died of AIDS and his widow proceeded to marry one if not more of his brothers (as each in turn died).

Because of the war in Northern Uganda, the situation of widows was particularly dire. For one thing, their numbers had understandably increased as families were dispersed and as male members had died, and for another, war-related land disputes had increased, and widows were often excluded. Formerly kidnapped women returning with children born in the bush could not identify a legitimate patrimony for their children. This left those children and their mothers without rights to land or, most critically, to its cultivation and use.

When a Northern Ugandan woman marries, she ordinarily moves into her husband's family's household. If her husband dies, she stands to lose her children (once they are no longer nursing) and the economic support of her husband's family. However, if her deceased husband's brother marries her, she will still have a place, as a second or third wife, and keep her children. Then, as part of her husband's extended family, she will continue to have access to land, her children will sometimes be given school fees, and she will retain the status of a married woman. On the other hand, if she is abandoned or sent away, a widow may have few economic options—one being to move to a trading center where she can brew beer and/or transact sex with men who drink there, or find a man who will marry her.

From this scenario, with or without widow inheritance, an HIV-positive widow can become a liability if she is sexually active. Given this possibility, it would be more beneficial for the society as a whole if a widow remains with her children and receives the support of her deceased husband's family. Frequently, I heard that the spread of HIV should be blamed on widows. Given that impoverished women transact sex for money or food to survive, it is reasonable to assume widows would transact sex for survival if ousted from familial support. In such stories, men have narratively disappeared.

The purpose of the story *Widow Inheritance* was to open up conversation around the multiple beliefs about, reasons for, and consequences of widow inheritance. At the same time I hoped participants, readers, and the audience would consider alternatives in light of this practice. Figure 3.1 shows a page from the

Figure 3.1

Mon Too

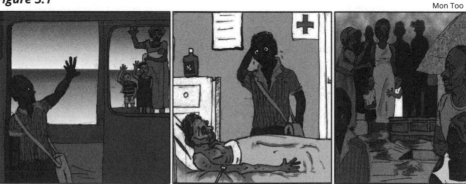

Odiko mere, Ogwal oyaa ipaco me wot neno ominere adit ma tye bedo itaun Lira.

Ogwal: Kong idong wunu aber.....abino dwogo paco iyonge nino moro anok.

Ikare ma Ogwal otuno bot ominere itaun me Lira, wie obin obale icawa ma oneno ominere pien kome ma onwongo obale atek pi kome ma onwongo tye alit. Omin Ogwal tye agoro ma dang pe twero kop.

beginning of *Widow Inheritance*, where the problems facing Ogwal and Santos, two brothers who have an older brother dying of AIDS, are presented. When the eldest brother dies, he leaves a widow, Akello, and two children.

How do public narratives interpret these problems?

I want the story to show how each person negotiates within trajectories of power and powerlessness. Relational transactions highlight absence of equivalency, and also the complicity among different characters (both men and women) to sustain this absence. In creating a composite narrative, one must create a story where vulnerability is not always explicated as automatic victimhood. One must be cautious not to lose narrative credibility by lumping victimization with social norms because these are not equivalent. While outsiders might look disapprovingly at a norm, the effect of the norm is quite different from its existence (Das 2000). Certainly not all inherited widows are victims. Without understanding this difference, a narrative about, for example, widow inheritance, would come out of the assumptions and perceptions of the viewer rather than the viewed: "the very gesture that appears to grant them recognition reduces them to what they are not—and often refuse to be—reifying their condition of victimhood while ignoring their history and muting their words" (Fassin 2012:254).

Suggesting that anyone who is inherited is a victim provokes misunderstandings and shame because in many cases being inherited with her children is a widow's preference and best option. For one thing, a widow might be more respected as an inherited wife than if she is driven away. While some widows are certainly victims of mistreatment, widow inheritance was a formerly respected cultural practice that has been egregiously affected by the AIDS epidemic and by war. Some readers might be critical that I am not mentioning gender rights or a woman's right to marital choice. However, in shaping a cultural narrative, I am creating a recognizable, complex reality, not a human rights treatise. Improved human rights might evolve as an outgrowth of a story like *Widow Inheritance*, but it is not the definitive focus of a narrative. The informational text for this story contained explanations of sexual and reproductive health rights and of sexual disease.

When creating the story *Widow Inheritance*, I learned that the public narrative often implied that a family should provide for the widow, that she should not be abandoned, or that a brother of the deceased should marry her. But because poverty and HIV infection have increased in Northern Uganda, behavior toward widows has changed (though not the public narrative), leading to their abandonment or mistreatment by the deceased husband's family, who sometimes blame the widow for her husband's death. This has increased problems for widows, their children, and the society as a whole.

Who are the central characters and how will their relations
and interactions heighten or reduce the problem?

The selection of appropriate characters and their interactions is essential to the credibility of a narrative. In the ethnographic data that led up to this story, I read interviews with and about brothers dying of AIDS and widows marrying surviving brothers. I heard about family and community pressure to marry a widow and about conflicts over ownership, rights, and access to a deceased brother's property, which would include the widow with her children if a brother marries her. On the other hand, if he does not marry her, his deceased brother's property might be distributed within the extended family or clan, without the widow and with or without her children. Therefore the brother who could inherit a widow stands to lose her property if he does not marry her. So in the story of widow inheritance, I needed brothers and their wives, widows, the extended family, neighbors, and children of the family as characters.

I wanted to show how the desires of story characters are set against the possibility of HIV transmission. This page from the story *Widow Inheritance* shows the second brother, Santos, complying with his parents' wishes to marry the widow, Akello. The parents tell Santos that it is a shame not to help his brother's widow. Meanwhile Santos's wife is privately telling her sister-in-law she does not want a co-wife, while her sister-in-law tells her she is obligated to accept her husband's decision (not shown). In the first panel of Figure 3.2, the family pressures Santos to marry Akello. In the last panel Santos is shown with the widow, Akello, and her children as he marries her as his second wife.

Figure 3.2

Mon Too

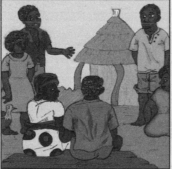 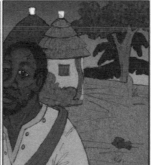 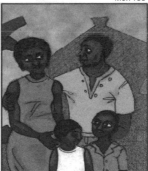

Aceng ki cware Ogwal omio onywal magi tam.

Aceng: Atat, ikobo wunu wod wu atidi ni myero wot lak dako ma bedo itaun ca. Gwok nyo kodi two ma oneko wod wu ca twero kobo ikom wod wu atidi kono.

Onywal: Kong inen kit ma dako man ki otino mere kom gi yot ki. Man nyutu ni kom gi kom pe lit atwali. Wod wa kom owalo ki yat pi kop me cato wilere omio otoo.

Awobi me aryo, Okello, oye me lako dako too ma ominere oweko. En okwanyo dako ni te dwoko itaun Lira.

Okello obin olako dako too pien itmare dako man onwongo cil totwal.

Okello: Abino gwoki ki neno ni otino ni ducu onwongo kony ma mite wek odong gini aber.

*What cultural events, encounters, beliefs, and practices
might directly or indirectly contribute to vulnerability?*

Central to *Widow Inheritance* are the funerals of the brothers (only the funeral of the
second brother is shown here), the gatherings where the family pressures a brother
to inherit a widow, and conversations where a current wife encounters a relative and
talks about her husband marrying a widow and how she feels about having a widow
as a co-wife. Cultural events and actions create credibility because they are empiri-
cally recognizable. Who in Northern Uganda does not recognize these events and
actions in their own lives or the lives of others in their communities? In the first
panel in Figure 3.3, the widow, Akello, is pregnant and the first wife of Santos is
clearly upset. Akello gives birth but shortly after that, Santos dies.

In Figure 3.4, the parents of the brothers are commiserating with Akello and
suggesting that she marry Ogwal, the youngest brother. In the last frame on this
page, Akello goes to Ogwal assuming he will marry her while the other widow of
Santos looks on.

*What is the logic of shame and silence in this
production of narrative vulnerability?*

The logic of shame is symbolized in how character relations and interactions expose
or hide failure and/or achieve pride. This is evident in the descriptive text and the dialogue of story characters. The descriptive text in the story *Widow Inheritance* tells us
about the death of each brother, and the character dialogue interprets these deaths.
Through character dialogue the logic of shame is produced and expanded upon.

Figure 3.3

Mon Too

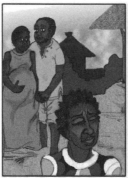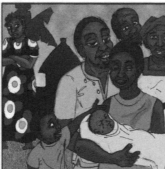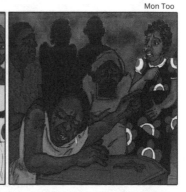

Iyonge nino moro anok, dako
alaka ma tye itaun ca te
bino paco kunu. Dako man
dong onwongo yac. Dako me
adwong kono yie pe obedo
ayom me neno nyeke ma tye
ayac.

Dako alaka obin onywalo
atin awobi. Yii jo paco ducu
onwongo yom atek pi atin man
nikwanyo ka Akullo, nyek dako
alaka man.

Lwak: Atin ma onywalo ni kome
tek totwal. Kong nen kit ma kok
ki. Kok idwon alongo.

Iyonge dwete abicel, atin adako
alaka te too oko. Dako man
okok ikom nyeke Akullo ni en
aye otyeto atinere omio otoo.

Figure 3.4

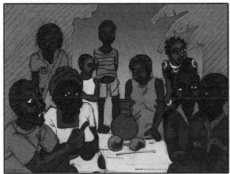 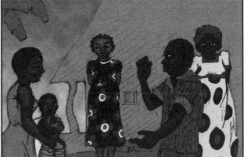

Iyonge dakika moro anok, Okello obin otoo oko idakatal kan ma onwongo en tye atwoye iye. En oweko mon aryo ka omedo ki dako ma en onwongo olako ca.

Onywal: Ogwal, omini en dong otoo oko ni ba! Yin myero ilak dako adwong kun omini atidi ni bino lako dako atidi wek omede wunu igwoko gi wek paco wa pe tur oko.

Awobi atidi obin oye lako dako atidi, ento Ogwal obin okwero lako dako ma omie oko.

Ogwal: An pe aye tam wu pien ka an alako dako adwong ca, an ki jo tura ducu twero bedo ma kom gi lit eka ate too bala omegi na aryo ma otoo ca.

Onywal: Ento dako adwong ca tye ma kome yot. Kong inen! pe dang maro butu piny atata. Kara ka pe iye gero, itamo ni nga ma twero lako dako nono te gwoko imiti a jo me paco ni.

What is not being talked about in this scenario of widow inheritance? Usually any wives of remaining brothers are neither asked nor allowed to give their opinions about whether their husband should marry his brother's widow. Many women object to widow inheritance, believing that a new co-wife might be HIV positive. I interviewed women who had been infected when a husband, unbeknownst to his wife, married a widow (not always the widow of his brother) as described by this respondent:

> Always there was fighting. There was chaos because when a new woman is brought, the old one is always neglected . . . now when there is a quarrel between my co-wife and I, now we sit down and try to resolve things peacefully or we ask others to help us if we can't solve it. From the program I learned that when a man wants to get a second wife, they should test their blood so that everyone knows their status because maybe her first husband died of AIDS and maybe the husband just brings her to his home without knowing her status. My husband just grabbed my co-wife. The co-wife, my husband, and I are infected and on medication. The training helped me to cope with life. . . . I think about my children and how they are going to live.

Another issue not openly discussed is what will happen to the widow's property. The brother of the deceased wants the widow's property and if he marries her, he will gain control of his dead brother's assets. However, if a widow refuses a brother who wants to marry her, she stands to lose her property and be chased away from her home. (For more about this, see the section about evaluation interviews in Chapter 5.)

In the story in these images, shown in Figure 3.5, Ogwal's parents say, "We have seen the widow and the children. They are very healthy!" Some still do not believe that one can look healthy and be HIV infected or they fear the consequences of a positive diagnosis. In denial, the parents are anticipating shame.

Ogwal decides not to inherit the widow, Akello, who is shamed because he has sexually rejected her. Therefore, one consequence of Ogwal's refusal to marry Akello is that she talks to Ogwal's wife, Aceng, and says that he has insulted her by refusing to marry her.

Akello also talks to Ogwal's sister and neighbors about his refusal to marry her. Groups of women in the community gossip about Aceng, saying she has bewitched her husband to prevent him from marrying Akello. Rather than appreciating Ogwal's decision, the community looks with disfavor at him and Aceng, his wife.

In what ways might this narrative project possibilities for change in conversations and actions?

When I am creating a narrative, I am not thinking about providing solutions in the story text. In a typical story, as part of the practice, program participants suggest alternative solutions after the story is read (Chapter 4, "The Pedagogy"). But occasionally I offer a possibility within the narrative plot itself in the voice of a story character. In *Widow Inheritance* I suggest a possible solution by having

Figure 3.5

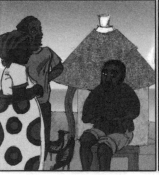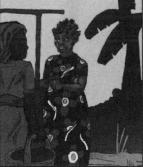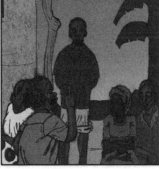

Iyonge nino anok, omin Ogwal aditere ni te too oko. Jo paco ducu okumu pi too man pien too man okunyo twon bur atut ipaco nono. Omin Ogwal otoo oweko dako acel ki otino kic adek. Iyonge onywal ki atekere obedo piny me neno ngo ma myero otim pi gwoko dako ki otino kic magi.

Onywal Ogwal: Wan tam wa tye ni, omin a too ma olube myero lak dako ma atoo oweko.

Ento dako omin gi me aryo okwero tam man acil kun kobo ni ka obedo amano twara eya ewoto oko.

Dako omin gi me aryo ca: Amina, an pe amito bedo imon nyek atwali.

Aceng: Cwari kom tye amito lako dako naca ba!

Jo paco obedo nyamo tam man karacel.

Onywal: Pe pore me dako a too ibedo abongo ngatoro igwoko. Otino mere obedo otino wa ma myero onwong yore me gwoko otino magi medo ki dako too ma wod wa oweko. Wod wa atidi ni myero wot bed Lira me konyo gwoko paco kunu ki gwoko otino.

Ogwal, the youngest brother, refuse to marry Akello. Instead he suggests that she stay in her house and that he will pay the school fees for her children (fig. 3.6). By saying he will not marry her, he is refusing to have sex with her. Paying school fees for children is an obligation usually assumed by the husband or the father of the children. In this act of apparent generosity, Ogwal is helping the widow and her children and protecting his family at the same time. Ogwal in turn will gain control of the widow's property, and Akello will cultivate land for Ogwal.

What activities in the pedagogic process—discussion questions, role-plays, and health information—might inform and transform the public narrative?

When creating a narrative, I think about questions and role-plays that will help participants explicate and interpret the narrative. Here is an example of the Discussion Questions and Role-Play Suggestions that follow the story, *Widow Inheritance*:

Group Questions for Critical Thinking and Dialogue for Widow Inheritance

1. What would you do if you were Ogwal? What advice would you give to Ogwal?
2. How would you end this story?
3. What do you think happened to Ogwal's brothers and his brother's wives?
4. Why did Santos marry his brother's widow?

Figure 3.6

Ododo ma tye Imung
Mon Too

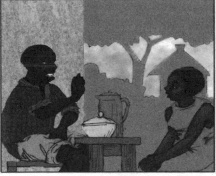 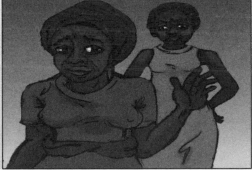

Dako too adwongere obino bot Ogwal kun kele dek amit ki mot. Dako man obwolo tam Ogwal wek yee lake pi bedo cware.

Ogwal: An gira abino culo pi kwan otino ni ducu. Abino neno ni agwoki ikit ma mite, ento pe abino laki me bedo cwari.

Ikare ma oneno ni tam Ogwal odoko tek, dako too man owoto bot dako Ogwal pi tamo ni kony kore me wek Ogwal gere wek bed gini mon nyek.

Dako too: Cwari onywara atek, aco atye amito ni en gera wek ogwok otino me kaka ni. An kena pe atwero gwoko otino ni. Kong ikop ki ba wek en lok tmare.

Aceng: Cwara Franko ka dong omoko tmare, nwongo dong omoko. Pe tye kit yore moro ma atwero kop ki eka te loko tmare.

5. How can Ogwal still help his brother's widow without hurting himself and his family?
6. What could Ogwal have said to prevent the death of Santos?
7. Why was Akello angry at Ogwal and at Aceng?
8. Why did Ogwal's parents believe the widows were in good health?
9. What could you say to Ogwal's parents or other people about the dangers of widow inheritance? How can people avoid these dangers?
10. What are good things about widow inheritance? What are bad things about it?

Role-Play Suggestions for Widow Inheritance

1. Ogwal and his parents discuss why Ogwal will not marry his brother's widow.
2. Ogwal and Aceng discuss why he will not marry her.
3. Ogwal and his parents discuss how to stop conflicts between husbands and wives.
4. Ogwal and his family discuss the dangers and benefits of widow inheritance.
5. Akello, Aceng, and their mother-in-law discuss the dangers and benefits of traditions like widow inheritance

Finally, I consider what kind of health information should follow a set of narratives. The story *Widow Inheritance* is grouped with stories related to HIV infection (Book 4 in the Uganda program). Book 4 contains factual information about STIs and HIV/AIDS. The images in Figure 3.7 are examples of such information, showing the symptoms of a sexually transmitted disease in women and comparing them with symptoms in men. For example, though the text is not shown here, for one image it describes that often women, unlike men, have no symptoms for an

Figure 3.7

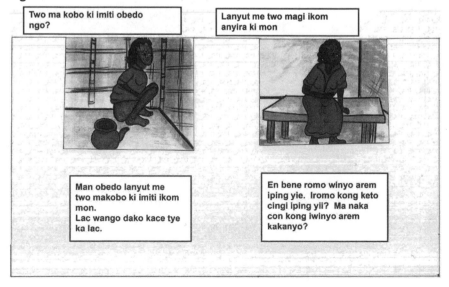

STI. Book 4 also provides pictorial and textual health information about the signs, symptoms, methods of transmission of STIs and HIV and AIDS in women and men, and about condoms and how to use them.

In the children's rights program, I included information about how to listen to and talk to children, how to help children when they have conflicts, and how to talk to youth about sexual and reproductive health. Figure 3.8 shows one page from a book in the children's rights program, about how adults can react when children fight.

In the environmental education program I included information about the water cycle, building walls to prevent erosion, planting trees, keeping markets clean, preventing water contamination, planting different crops, using natural pesticides, and composting, among other environmental information. Figure 3.9 shows one page from the informational text about the water cycle.

Figure 3.8

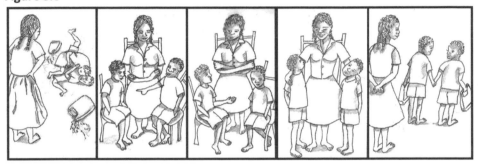

Figure 3.9

Ki sa sik dlo a ye?

Sik Dlo a

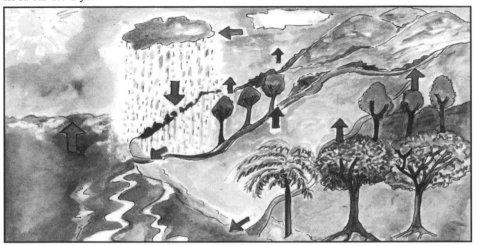

Gade imaj sa ki gen sik dlo a. Ki sa ou wè la? Sa k ap pase nan imaj sa ? Poukisa pyebwa yo enpòtan pou lavi nou epi pou lavni nou ?

Data analysis and plot design essential components in the creation of narrative practice, require one to think about what the data shows and how it can be formed into a composite story plot. Part of analyzing data is considering how questions, role-plays, and information will enhance and expand the impact of the narratives. The composite narrative and the informational text must be congruent in purpose. Narrative structure is another consideration crucial to the creation of a composite narrative, which will be covered in the next Step 3.

Step 3: Structuring the Composite Narrative

We live contradictions—some causing constant misery, others offering ways out without disrupting others' expectations of us. I was interviewing a young, energetic woman who is a third wife. She explained her husband: "He is an old man who only lasts a few minutes." She talked about her initial sadness after her marriage to him. "He treated me well, but I was so frustrated . . . so miserable. I was ashamed of my life." Then she met the old man's younger brother. They fell in love. She told me that she has two children with the younger brother. "We are happy," she laughed, not with malice but with grace.

I asked her, "Will you ever tell the old man?"

"Oh, no, no! That would hurt his feelings. I could never do that! He is so good to me. He is happy because he believes that he fathered two sons. You know they look like him." She had managed to please everyone including herself. She was able to fulfill her public and affinal obligations while living a fulfilling under-story. Not everyone I interview is so lucky.

Contradictions that Cause, Sustain, and Reinforce Shame and Vulnerabilities

In each story central characters feel shame in their interactions with others. "Shame is what is produced in the absolute concomitance of subjectification and desubjectification, self-loss and self-possession, servitude and sovereignty" (Agamben 1999:107).

The question for me is how will shame be articulated in the narrative structure? In order to narratively depict shame, I create dialectical oppositions between a person and a context, between the private and the public, between the internal and the external. As I read through the data and decide on the central theme of a story, contradictions become apparent. In each story, the characters desire love, protection, social acceptance and approval, and the promise of happiness. However, in the hidden text, things go awry and desires are subverted, nullified, or not achieved.

I have chosen three stories from three different programs to explain how narrative plot structure develops and mirrors shame. From the African American project, the story *Mama You Don't See Me* explores the contradictions between a child's desire for love and the subversion of these desires by her stepfather, a child molester. From the Latino project, the story *Who Is This Man I Thought I Loved?* examines the conflict between a woman's expectations for an understanding, loving husband and her reality of a jealous, abusive one. From the Ugandan project, the story *Girl Child* considers the familial need to have a male heir set against a husband's rejection of his wife because she has only given birth to girls, further contrasted with his wife's desire for social acceptance for her girl children and for herself.

Vulnerabilities that Increase in Intensity Over Time

In each story, whether about child abuse, domestic violence, or preference for boy children, the degree of vulnerability increases over time. In the story *Mama You Don't See Me*, the child molester, Raymond, becomes more invasive and demanding toward the child, Dee. At the same time, Raymond convinces Dee that he loves her and is protecting her from a world that does not understand her. He pits Dee against her mother. As Dee becomes more sexually provocative with boys her own age (since this is how she values herself), she gets into trouble at school. This escalates hostility between Dee and her mother and reinforces Raymond's hold over Dee. While Dee's mother increasingly refuses to give Dee the comfort and attention she needs, the molester increasingly indulges her.

In the story *Who Is This Man I Thought I Loved?*, a young woman named Claudia who lives in Mexico marries a Latino day laborer named Raul who lives in Los Angeles. After their marriage, Raul brings Claudia to Los Angeles. Because her English is poor, he informs Claudia how she should dress and act in urban America. Raul believes that she wants to socialize, seek work, learn English, and hang out with a "promiscuous" woman friend because he believes Claudia desires other men. Raul's physical and emotional abuse of Claudia intensifies over time in tandem with his increasing jealousy. Claudia makes up excuses to her friends when they see bruises on her face. After each beating, Raul, when sober, apologizes for his behavior and asserts his love for and desire to protect Claudia.

In the Ugandan story *Girl Child*, a young man named Adur marries Adong, and for two years she does not give birth. Adur's family is critical of Adong because she is barren, but eventually she becomes pregnant and gives birth to twin girls. Criticism from Adong's mother-in-law and other women increases, but Adur assures Adong that she will give birth to a baby boy and secretly visits a traditional healer to get herbal treatments. Adong becomes pregnant, but again she gives birth to a baby girl. Her mother- and father-in-law put pressure on Adur to take a second wife that they find for him, but Adong does not want Adur to do this. In his anger at Adong for her failure to give birth to a son, he begins to abuse her. After Adur takes a second wife and she gives birth to a boy, Adur's abuse of Adong intensifies.

Each story captures the significance of shame in the intensification of shame-provoking interactions between story characters.

Forces that Lessen Shame and Vulnerability

The composite narratives are not characterizations of vulnerability that ignore forces that work toward reducing shame. I want to avoid creating characters as frozen binary examples of good versus evil (though in a few instances this is difficult to avoid). In reality things are not that simple. Achieving dialogue between program participants will be difficult during the pedagogical activities (Chapter 4, "The Pedagogy"), if the story characters represent extremes. The most successful stories have multiple possibilities for transactions between story characters and therefore, multiple possibilities for participant discussion as well.

In each story, vulnerable characters have choices, though sometimes quite limited ones. Characters take action to live with, reduce, or end their feelings of shame. Sometimes forces act to alleviate a character's feelings of shame, but sometimes healing or helping forces are submerged or overwhelmed by powerful destructive ones. In each narrative, story characters transact their lives amidst these forces.

In the story *Mama You Don't See Me*, at first Dee's grandfather is her protector. When Dee's mother and grandmother are critical of Dee's behavior, the grandfather listens to and supports her. When her grandfather dies, Dee has lost her protector and her sexual abuse heightens. Dee contemplates suicide, and Angel, Dee's confidant, tries to dissuade her. When Angel and Dee are adults, Angel helps Dee reflect on past experiences and think about how Dee will protect her own child in the future.

In the story *Who Is This Man I Thought I Loved?*, Claudia develops a friendship with a neighbor, Angel, who helps her find employment. Angel also tells her to call 911 in case of emergency, because Angel suspects Raul is abusing Claudia. Claudia's employer offers her the chance to take English lessons. Each instance of help leads to another hurtful encounter with Raul as he accuses Claudia of using her friendships, English lessons, and employment as a means to meet men.

In the story *Girl Child*, Adong marries and moves from her natal village into her husband's village. At different points in the story Adong seeks the support of her husband, Adur, who assures her she will give birth to a boy. Adong secretly consults a traditional healer for advice and herbs. In two instances Adong goes to her parents for help. Her father gives her money to pay for school fees for her children if she promises to return to her husband.

Structural and Textual Narrative Transactions

In a culturally credible narrative, story characters function within the harnesses imposed by culture and circumstance. Interpersonal transactions are woven within descriptive and dialogic text. In the story *Mama You Don't See Me*, when Raymond first molests Dee, he offers her a pizza (which Dee's mother has refused her). This is the first episode of molestation. As the sexual demands of Raymond increase, the negotiations between Dee and Raymond intensify. Dee is growing up and she is learning the art of manipulation from her sexual predator, Raymond. Raymond transacts sexual access to Dee in exchange for the new clothes he purchases for her.

In the story *Who Is This Man I Thought I Loved?*, Claudia is invited to cook for a party. Claudia wants to be a "good" wife, but she unintentionally imperils herself when she attends the party and socializes with the other partygoers. After the party, Raul accuses Claudia of flirting with men at the party and beats her. Later when Claudia misses a bus because her employer is showing her an ad for English lessons, Raul beats Claudia and throws the announcement for English lessons away. Claudia is privately looking for a way out. However, when she is faced with ending the abuse, she fears the loss of what she perceives to be her only security.

In the story *Girl Child*, Adur's parents are able to negotiate a second wife for him because his first wife has given birth only to girls. Interactions between Adong and Adur become more abusive as time goes on because Adong, in Adur's mind, has failed to live up to her marital obligation. Adur becomes infatuated with his second wife who has borne him a son. Adong negotiates for the education of her daughters, but Adur is negotiating for an end to their schooling because, as he says, "They are girls." Adur rejects his obligation because Adong has failed in her obligation to him. Desire motivates character negotiation, but Adur has the backing of culture, of society, which sees Adong's failure to produce a male child as a collective and familial loss.

Juxtaposing Descriptive and Dialogic Forces

In each composite story I create dialectic tension between two opposing narrative forces: the public *top-stories* and the private and secret *under-stories*. When I began developing narrative practice, I embedded these transactions in the narrative. But as I became more aware of their significance to the readers and the pedagogy, I set them up as separate, distinct subtexts by highlighting their appearances.

Both the top-stories and the under-stories are culturally patterned. The top-story is narrative-appearance, the commonplace interpretation of what we collectively feel and believe. It is what we publicly acknowledge—the acceptable, openly lived story of our common sensibilities. The top-story socially affirms, defines, and reinforces beliefs about who we are.

In the narrative plot structure, the top-story is juxtaposed against the under-story. The under-story is forbidden, hidden, and shameful. It defies public obligation and expectation as well as undermining the pomp and pretense of characters in the top-story. The top-story is what others want us to know about them, while the under-story is what others do not want us to know, a collectively agreed upon narrative-disappearance.

Powerlessness is often veiled in unspeakable under-stories, sub-narratives that invoke the origins of vulnerabilities and how they are lived. Knowing and speaking the under-story can be socially powerful or debilitating, conciliatory or confrontational. We learn about each other from the under-story, a suspected truth that, until its unveiling, deflects public conversation and comparison. Under-stories have multiple consequences, ranging from the mild and inconsequential to the horrific and devastating. Like the public story, the under-story is commonplace and patterned because the under-story is the hidden text in everyone's sight.

Narratively and in reality, neither the top-story nor the under-story can exist or thrive without the other. In their interrelatedness I create dialectical tension. As an example, a person who is socially stigmatized, let us say as an HIV carrier, retains social disfigurement in an agreed upon public narrative that he or she is dangerous. At the same time, his or her self-shame is experienced in the loss of him or herself in this public objectification or stigmatization. Being an HIV carrier is a loss of the other—the other being the possibility for unbiased interactions, social acceptance, and affiliations.

The juxtaposition of these two related sub-narratives sets the stage for contradiction. As Roland Barthes states, "Who endures contradiction without shame?" (1975:3) As contradictions are encountered, story characters experience transgression and so does the audience—if the story authentically mirrors a reconstructed reality. Textual transactions create narrative plot and structure recognizable to the culturally similar audience. I will give examples of these transactions in excerpts from these three stories.

Excerpts from a Narrative from the African American Program

Figure 3.10 shows scenes early in the story *Mama You Don't See Me*. Dee's mother and grandmother chastise Dee for talking with a neighbor and playing with boys on her way home from church. Raymond, her stepfather, tries to assert fatherly authority, but Dee replies that he is not her father so he should not be telling her what to do. As the story opens, the reader sees Dee's childlike playfulness. For the reader, this childlikeness will reinforce the profound loss of the self that Dee will experience in the impending under-stories. In this first under-story, shown in Figure 3.11, Raymond is alone with Dee. As soon as Dee's mother leaves, Raymond colludes with Dee to order a pizza against Dee's mother's wishes.

The images in Figures 3.10 and 3.11 juxtapose the top- and under-story in the first incidence of child molestation. *Mama You Don't See Me* is a retrospective narrative about an adult woman's interpretation of her childhood. Blue is the color of memory. When the story switches to the present, it is fully colored.

In Figure 3.12, Dee begins to lie and get into trouble at school. Dee's grandfather tries to comfort her though Dee's mother says that he is spoiling her. The

Figure 3.10

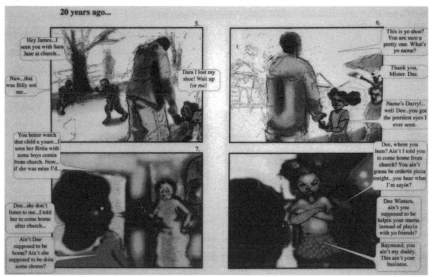

Figure 3.11

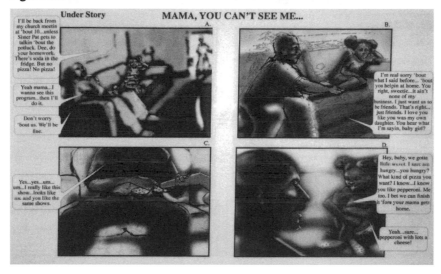

antagonism of Dee's mother is set against the friendship of her grandfather. Later the reader sees Dee flirting with boys at her school and being solicited by a neighbor, the same neighbor who in a previous image "kindly" handed Dee her shoe after she lost it playing with friends.

In the next under-story, shown in Figure 3.13, Raymond's sexual abuse intensifies. Then, in the top-story, Figure 3.14, Dee and Raymond go on a shopping trip because Raymond sees that Dee is jealous of her new baby sister and recognizes a chance to ingratiate himself with her. Dee's mother accuses Raymond of spoiling

Figure 3.12

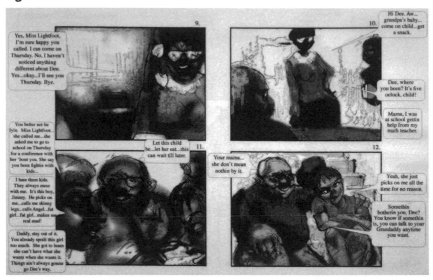

Figure 3.13

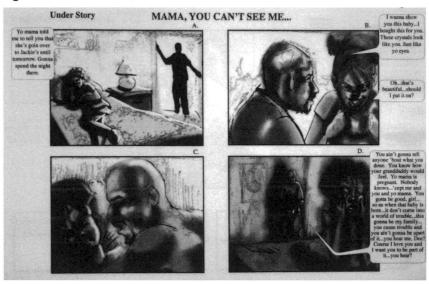

Dee by buying her clothes instead of clothes for the baby. The reader sees how Raymond manipulates Dee and her mother to build an alliance with Dee and at the same time pit her and her mother against each other. As Dee experiences the loss of her mother's love and protection, she is in effect losing herself.

From the initial interviews, respondents said they were molested as children in part because their mother's desire for a husband made her blind to the abuse of her child. When the child acted badly, the mother perceived this as an obstacle to this desire. Respondents also said they believed their mother had been molested as a child, which led to this blindness.

Figure 3.14

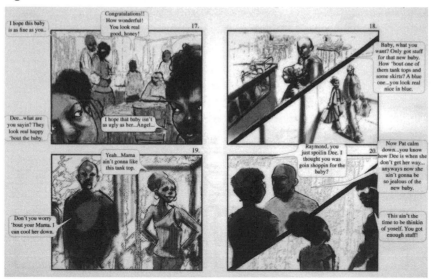

Excerpts from a Narrative from the Latino Program

Narratives in the Latino project focus on the life and circumstances of undocumented Latino immigrants living in Los Angeles. In the story *Who Is This Man I Thought I Loved?*, the top-story and under-story are juxtaposed in increasingly violent episodes. The episode shown in Figure 3.15 occurs after Claudia and Raul attend a party. At the party, Claudia tells Raul he should not drink too much. On their walk home, Raul is angry that Claudia interfered with his drinking and accuses her of flirting with men at the party.

The first image of the under-story, shown in Figure 3.16, is the same as an image in the top story. In subsequent frames the under-story is different than the top story. I experimented with this structure in order to show how the top-story could, in part, be read independent of the under-story and still make sense. I thought this kind of structuring would emphasize how domestic violence can

Figure 3.15   *Figure 3.16*

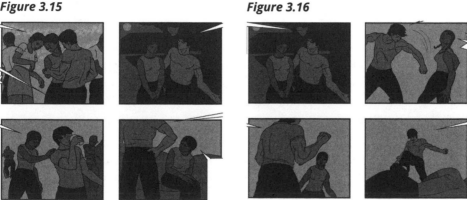

Figure 3.17   *Figure 3.18*

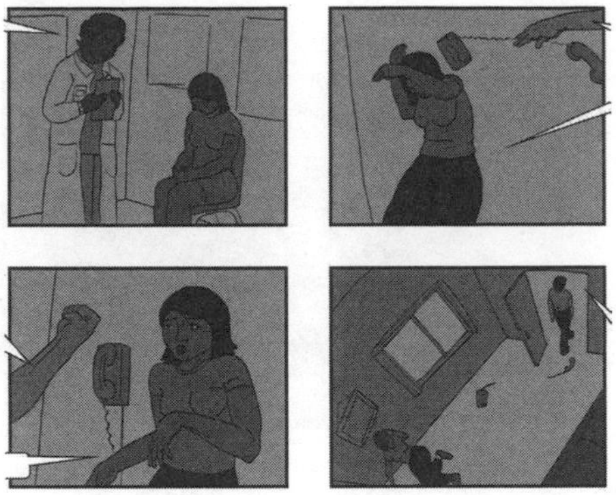

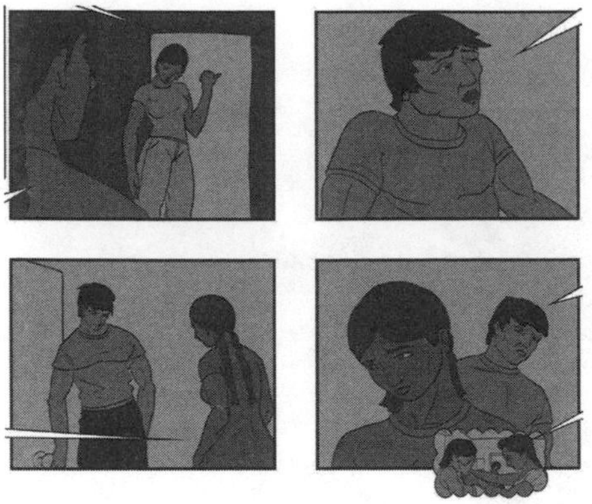

easily be hidden by outward appearances. Here Raul calls Claudia a whore and trash and says, "What would my parents think if they knew what you were doing. You think you can flirt with men and think I don't know what you're doing?"

The story progresses and Raul's abuse heightens. In Figure 3.17, a friend, Angel, encourages Claudia to meet her at a mall. Raul tells Claudia that Angel has a bad reputation so Claudia should not hang around with her. In the next images Raul apologizes, though without the under-story (not shown), Raul's abuse would be unknown to the reader.

In Figure 3.18 Claudia feels unwell. At a clinic, a doctor tells Claudia that she has gonorrhea and that she needs to tell her husband. When Claudia tries to explain the diagnosis to Raul, he accuses her of being a whore, rips the phone from the wall and leaves. This is the third of five under-stories in the story of Claudia and Raul.

Excerpts from a Narrative from the Ugandan Program

Narratives in the Ugandan program focus on Northern Ugandans (who had experienced a twenty-three-year war), particularly on domestic, sexual, and civil violence, and cultural practices which can increase vulnerabilities. In *Girl Child*, Adong has given birth to female twins and is being harassed by her mother-in-law and neighbors. In this first image, Adong's husband, Adur, appears to be showing support for his wife against community pressure (fig. 3.19). Later in this story Adur will succumb to this pressure. Because of her feelings of shame, Adong tries to change her situation. After hearing her mother-in-law's suggestion that Adur take a second wife (fig. 3.20), Adong seeks out a traditional healer to obtain herbal medicine so that she can produce a male child (fig. 3.21). This is the under-story, as going to a traditional healer is a shameful act and something Adong would not want Adur or others to know.

People say traditional healers sometimes have sex with women clients or provide them with herbs and secret incantations directed at a person's sexual behavior.

Figure 3.19

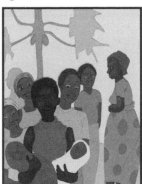

Figure 3.20

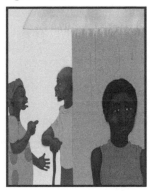

Figure 3.21

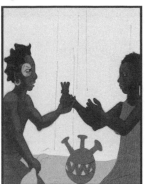

These are believed to have magical or medicinal consequences to achieve the desired effect. One desired effect for women is to control men's sexuality, as it is believed a man's ability to have sex with other women can be influenced by a healer's remedies. If this is the case, a man will only be able to have sex with the woman who is doing the "magic," which is not necessarily what the man in question desires. Men also seek the help of traditional healers for problems with female partners for similar reasons. Healers' remedies and advice generally address sexual and reproductive issues including infidelity, impotence, and infertility.

In the top-story, Adong becomes pregnant but again she gives birth to a girl. In the under-story, Adong refuses sex with Adur because she wants to calm their crying baby girl. He tells her to ignore the baby because it is only a baby girl, but Adong refuses and Adur hits her (fig. 3.22). In the next frame, Adong hears her mother-in-law commenting on the hips of a woman and how she would produce sons for their family (fig. 3.23).

Adong seeks help from her parents, but when she returns to her husband, she sees her possessions have been put outside of her house (fig. 3.24). Another woman is sweeping the compound. Adur has taken a second wife. Before long, the second wife produces a son.

Figure 3.22

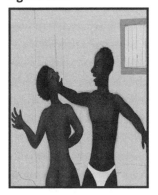

Figure 3.23

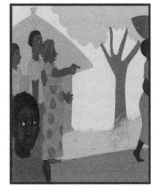

Figure 3.24

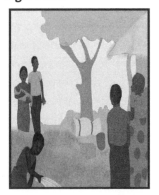

Figure 3.25   *Figure 3.26*

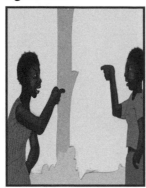   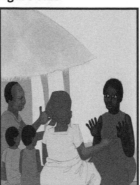

In the under-story, Figure 3.25, the second wife is telling Adong that Adong does not please their husband and that is why Adur does not visit or stay with her. She tells Adong to stop complaining, because there is not enough food or money for her daughters' education or for Adong's expectations. Adong's third baby girl dies because no one gives Adong money to take the baby to the hospital (not shown). The story continues.

Adur is not providing school fees for his daughters. In the under-story (not shown), Adong and Adur argue, and she tells him she needs money for school fees for their twin daughters. He tells her that the girls do not need to go to school because soon they will marry. Adong says she will go back to her parents, and Adur tells her to go because she is useless. The next image, Figure 3.26, shows Adong visiting her parents. They tell her that she should be patient because a man usually comes back to his first wife. But Adong tells them she does not want Adur as a husband anymore because he does not pay school fees. Adong's father agrees to pay school fees if she goes back to her husband. In the next under-story (not shown), Adong steals money from Adur so that she can send her daughters to school.

Top-Stories and Under-Stories in Narrative Practice

The juxtaposition of the top- and under-story in the narrative text and structure is essential to narrative practice. When I juxtapose the top-story and the under-story, I am setting up relational paradox. In each story, the under-story is a source of shame because it sets the characters up against what is socially desired and desirable. In the public performance of the characters in the top-story, they are deflecting the frustration and subversion of the under-story. In the story about child molestation, when Dee is flirting with boys or fighting with her mother, she is acting out her desire for friendship and attention that her private world has subverted. In the story about domestic violence, when Claudia is enjoying a party or trying to go out with a friend, she is trying to create a semblance of normalcy and friendship set against the private abuse of her husband. In the story about preference for boy children, when Adong goes to a traditional healer, seeks the support of her parents, and advocates for her daughter's education against her husband's wishes, she is trying to protect her children and herself from abandonment and discrimination.

Important to the juxtaposition of the top- and under-story is how, why, and in what ways transactions take place within and between the top- and under-story. Transactions in the text are also taking place within the structure of the narrative. This not only illuminates the suffering and demise of characters, it but also shows how characters endure and manage their circumstances. When participants see how a child molester manipulates a child, they witness how a vulnerable child manipulates the world in order to accommodate her powerlessness. When participants see how a husband physically abuses his wife, they also witness how his wife tries to work and learn English while managing her husband's accusations and beatings. When participants see how a community discriminates against a woman because she has not produced a son, they also witness how this woman copes with the discrimination toward her children and herself. This woman persists in getting school fees so that her daughters can continue in school. She is living within the harnesses of a community that has rejected her because she has not fulfilled a cultural requirement and because her daughters are an unwanted burden to the family.

Narrative transactions invoke reflexive shame felt in the experience of characters' social- and self-loss. Whether an HIV carrier, an abused child, or a woman who has not given birth to a son, the person shamed fears exposure. The public narrative sustains fear of exposure because of a publicly agreed-upon top-story that sufficiently silences the shame-filled under-story. According to Pierre Bourdieu, our social dispositions are etched on the template of the self (1990). However, shame can be a force that can reorder this template and move the self to other possibilities (Probyn 2005).

In the narratives, power and powerlessness are felt in the structuring of emerging, suppressed, and subverted desires and in the shaping of negotiations within both open and concealed plights. As the characters move in and between the top- and under-texts, the audience witnesses what those characters are experiencing. While the participants observe and hear how characters transact their lives, they reflect on their own or others experiences in doing the same. This achieves narrative believability critical to this practice. Credibility is also achieved in how each narrative is contextualized in voice and imagery, which I will talk about in the next step.

Step 4: Narrative Contextualization

> The language! It's our life. It comes to an understanding of what's real . . . it's how everybody talks. That's why they listen to it, 'cause they lived through it. If you say, "the doctor said this and that," that's a boring, sad-ass program . . . that's what they're gonna to be sayin.' But when you're talkin' the same language, the same way we live,

who's gonna say it ain't true? "I thought what you thought" . . . "I'm
gonna quit doin' it" . . . "it's on the streets" . . . that's what's came
outta their mouths 'cause it ain't shit when we was out there, and we
couldn't say it 'cause we was right out there doin' it.
—*participant from the African American project 2005*

Text and imagery articulate interactions and emotions in the composite narratives.
There are two types of text in the narratives: descriptive and dialogic. The descriptive text is written in the third person, describing setting, time, place, and actions.
Descriptive text moves the plot forward. This text is written within the facilitators'
manuals, which they read to participants during each learning session. The dialogic text is written in the first person and is in both the facilitators' manuals and
participants' books.

The descriptive text is explanatory, but the dialogic text is affective, more connected to emotions, and therefore more closely tied to an individual's recognition
of an experience. Character dialogue triggers memory. I heighten the engagement
of listeners by using dialogue that will evoke recollections of vivid and intense
human interactions. These will excite participants' emotions.

The purpose of the narratives is to influence what people say and how they
speak. When participants listen to story characters, they get ideas about what they
themselves might have said or not said in similar circumstances, and how verbal
exchanges between story characters led to conflict or compromise.

All the stories are translated into the participants' everyday language. In order
to accomplish this, I find (as I explained in the first step) translators who are well
versed in the local vernacular. I also ask translators to translate interviews word
for word. These translations sound odd in English but they give me a richer sense
of how people use words and phrases metaphorically. Word-for-word translation
helps me understand culturally meaningful dialogue, and because of this, it helps
me to create this dialogue between story characters. I am interested in idiomatic
expressions with shock value—phrases that people might say privately in emotional conflicts, or phrases a reader or audience would react to because these are
not ordinarily uttered in public discourse.

When analyzing data (Step 2) from the ethnographic interviews, I highlight
repetitive words and conversations. I extract these from the interviews so I can use
them to create character dialogue in the stories. During an ethnographic interview,
the interviewer asks respondents to repeat what was actually said in a critical situation. When I review the data, I hear repetitive patterns of speech being used by
people in conflictive situations. These patterns may not reflect everyone's conversations, but they represent normative discourse—culturally significant exchanges
that the audience will immediately recognize.

I use recognizable cultural metaphors in character dialogue. For example,
when English-language speakers say "I have butterflies in my stomach," there is a

shared cultural meaning not necessarily familiar to non-native English speakers. In Uganda, when a woman angrily says to her husband, "I'm not going to feed your anus," this phrase resonates with participants. When a story character says it, participants respond with laughter and approval because it carries meanings that everyone recognizes but which are not normally heard in a public forum. Walter Benjamin wrote, "To articulate the past historically does not mean to recognize it the way it really was. It means to seize hold of a memory as it flashes up at a moment of danger" (1968:257).

That is, using a phrase such as "I'm not going to feed your anus" in a public setting evokes the danger of the unexpected, igniting memories of crisis to the audience or readers.

Character dialogue is more than a reflection of a situation; it is in fact the situation itself (Holquist 1990). Therefore, in this regard, character dialogue must exactly replicate what the audience has known and heard. When interviewing Ugandans, for instance, they tell me that infertility is a serious problem. When women describe the abuse they suffer if infertile, I ask them what was said to them and how they responded. They tell me a mother-in-law or husband might say, "You are nothing but a toilet." This metaphorically compares the infertility of a wife to a waste repository, saying she consumes but produces nothing of value. The speaker is asserting that the infertile woman is a waste to the household into which she married. Later, when writing a story about a woman who has not given birth, I incorporate this expression into the dialogue between an anxious, shamed wife and her disappointed, equally shamed husband, who is being pressured by his family to divorce and remarry or take a second wife.

Similarly, the title of the story *I Took an Animal from the Road, So I Will Return It to the Road* is taken from a Haitian Creole expression that metaphorically describes the power of the caregiver over the powerlessness of the child, the extreme differences in their statuses, and the ironic "benevolence" of the caregiver. Comparing the child to an animal (without conscience or will) gives justification for the cruel treatment by the caregiver. Expressions like these trigger immediate recognition. In the context of a publicly read narrative, they also provoke shame: *Who has heard this expression and remained quiet?* And worse still, *who has said it?*

I rework and repeat common phrases that have particular cultural salience in order to reinforce the story plot and intention. Symbolic repetition is critical to spoken and literary text (Aristotle 1954). This repetition occurs in overlapping meanings reiterated in character conversation and imagery. In the Haitian children's rights program, I used the common phrase "she is there for that" and reworked it as the title of one story, *Is This What She Is For?* This phrase implies that the purpose of a child in servitude is to fulfill the sexual desires and needs of young men in the household. At the end of this story, when the child in servitude, Josette (now a young woman), is pregnant, the two brothers of the household repeat this phrase by saying, "I had her once. Isn't this what she is here for?"

In the story *Mama, You Don't See Me*, from the African American Program, I reiterated the significance of the title in different contexts within the story. In Figure 3.27, at the end of the story, the main character, Dee, is talking to her friend Angel, expressing her feelings about her memory of sexual abuse:

Figure 3.27

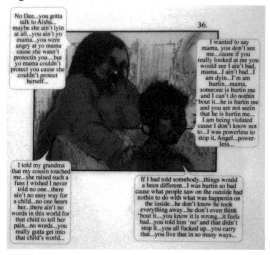

> *I wanted to say "Mama . . . you don't see me . . . 'cause if you really looked at me you would see I ain't bad, Mama. . . . I ain't bad. . . . I am dyin,' Mama. . . . I am hurtin.' Mama, someone is hurtin' me, and I can't do nothin' 'bout it. He is hurtin' me and you are not seein' that he is hurtin' me. I am being violated 'cause I don't know not to." I was powerless to stop it, Angel, powerless. . . .*

I build empathy by showing the complications of shame and how it results in risk to others as well as to the person being shamed. Some of the stories describe how people, because of shame, are being infected with HIV or are infecting others. The stories do not blame, but show circumstances that increase risk, often without the knowledge of those being exposed.

I use language to connote prejudices and misunderstanding. In the African American story *If I Revealed Myself, Would I Be Cast Off?*, a schoolteacher finds out she is HIV infected. At the same time, the teacher develops an empathetic relationship with a gay student. The story of the schoolteacher, whose husband is on the down-low, is told in tandem with a story of a gay high school student. Neither the husband nor the gay student can openly express their sexuality because they fear humiliation.

In this excerpt from Figure 3.28, the student is claiming he has a girlfriend, while the preacher exhorts his parishioners into a homophobic perspective—a perspective not uncommon in the African American communities where the ethnographic research was conducted.

> *Now we gotta problem . . . we got a big problem in this country. We got men marrying men . . . women marrying women. We got a problem. If God had meant it to be that way, it would be Adam and Steve . . . not Adam and Eve. We are going against the Word . . . the Word of the Bible . . . our Father, our dear Lord left us the B-I-B-L-E . . . Basic Instructions Before Leaving Earth.*

Figure 3.28

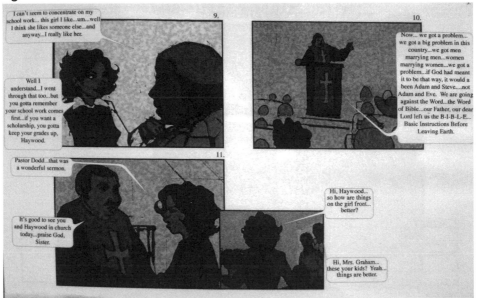

In this story there are multiple risks: first, there is risk of HIV transmission to women whose partners also have unprotected sex with men, and second, there is risk for gay people who do not have family and community acceptance and therefore hide their sexuality and behavior. The high numbers of incarcerated African American men and their frequent appearances and disappearances in communities where heterosexuality is the norm and homosexuality is frowned upon (as the preacher relates) increases everyone's risks. Regardless of whether a man self-identifies as a homosexual, men who have been incarcerated and experienced male-to-male sex while in prison might continue having sex with men clandestinely after leaving prison while at the same time being publicly sexually identified with women.

— ♦ —

In the story *Victoria's Secret* (from the Latino project), about a transgender Latino, Victor's father arrives home drunk when Victor is washing dishes with his mother (fig. 3.29). The father threatens to beat the mother if she does not stop treating Victor like a girl.

In one of the under-stories, Victor secretly tries on a dress and jewelry. His mother finds these things and accuses the father of having another woman. Victor tries to stop his parents from fighting and admits that the dress and jewelry belong to him (fig. 3.30). At this point, his father says, "You are a man! Not a woman! If ever I see you dressed up in women's clothes, I will kill you! I will kill you! Do you understand, Victor?"

Finally, in desperation, Victor's mother takes Victor to a doctor. The doctor represents a medically correct and compassionate view:

Figure 3.29

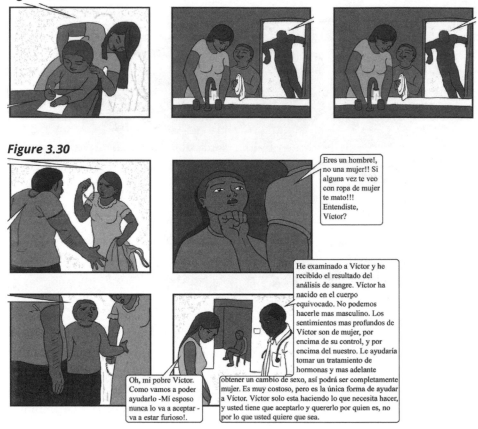

Figure 3.30

I examined Victor and completed some tests. Victor is not sick. He does not suffer from a disease. Victor feels that he is female, but as we know, his outer body is male. We do not know why this happens. Some believe it is biological . . . some that it is psychological, but again . . . we don't know. What we do know is that this is how Victor feels and we must respect his feelings. There are medical advances now that can help Victor.

The doctor goes on to assure Victor's mother that she has not done anything wrong. He says, "I know you are a good mother because you saw that your son needed help and you are trying to help him." Then he says, "Imagine how you would feel if people told you that you were not a woman, but that you were a man and now you must behave as a man. Then you might get some idea of how society makes Victor feel." He asks Victor's mother to bring Victor's father to the office because the doctor wants to explain these things to him.

Victoria's Secret is a narrative about a Latino woman at risk of HIV infection because her husband is engaging in unprotected sex with transgender women. I also created an empathetic story of a transgender woman alongside the story of a wife who acquires an STI from her husband—because the wife and the transgender woman are having unprotected sex with the same man. As pointed out earlier, the HIV prevalence in Los Angeles of transgender Latinos was high. From the interviews I learned that, while transgender respondents were telling me that they ordinarily had unprotected sex with married Latino men, married Latinas were telling me their husbands had requested unprotected anal sex with them.

Characters engage in dialogic interactions that establish their vulnerabilities. The Ugandan project focuses on the sexual and reproductive health vulnerabilities of Northern Ugandans. Most Northerners had experienced the consequences of a twenty-three-year war instigated by the Lord's Resistance Army. When I conducted research (2004), the war was still going on, but by the time I implemented the program (2010-2012), the war had ceased. In 2010, people were experiencing harsh conditions living in IDP camps, unable to return to their homes because their homes had either been burned or their land was under dispute. The story *Temporary Soldiers* is set in a refugee camp. The desires of impoverished girls living in the camps and selling small items to make money are set against the desires of soldiers with money. A child seller, impressed by the things other young sellers are being given by soldiers, wishes she had the attentions of a soldier. Later, a soldier entices the child seller into his house on the pretext of paying her money he owes her. There he rapes her. The dialogue in Figure 3.31 shows how the soldier cultivates the child's trust, desires, and attention. He says, "Here are money and a gift for the pancakes and the mangoes."

In the third frame, the same soldier says, "You are a good girl. You must be careful here because there are men in the camps who treat girls badly."

The soldier implies that he is of good character because he is protective of the seller. This dialogue is in stark contrast to the later rape scene. One facilitator, after reading the story, became quite agitated, describing how this exact story happened to her niece. In her description the child had been encouraged into a relationship with a soldier because he had money. The participant was angry because after her

Figure 3.31

Mamaingaya Pola

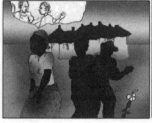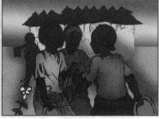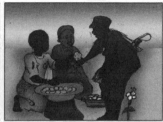

Nyako acel: Aceng ka ibedo wire icuk kan ogati ni pe awile. Wot icat ogati ni bot omony.

Nyako okene: Omony maro wilo ogati ibot wa kare ikare. Icel icel dang ka cente me aloka pe, ojali naka cente ame myero odwok oko.

Awot Aceng: Ineno jami na ni, atambara kede nyor inguta ni, awota moro ame obedo amony aye omia.

Aceng: Anyira okene kori gi igum ateni. Inwongo awoti ame wilo jami abeco piri gire,

Amony: Gam cente me culo baya ogati anen agamo. Cente odong iwie nono pe dang idwogo. Ter iwot imi mama ni wek en konyere kede.

Figure 3.32

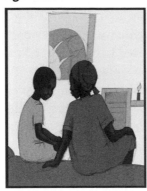

Figure 3.33

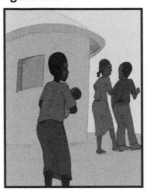

Figure 3.34

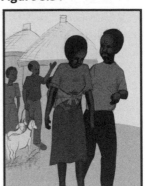

niece became pregnant, the soldier abandoned her. In chilling ways, war exacerbates inequities as normal desires can be so easily exploited.

Another story from the Uganda program, *Agnes*, story opens with a mother talking to her daughter about why it is important to avoid unprotected premarital sex. In Figure 3.32, the mother, Agnes, recounts how she became pregnant as a girl. She explains that after her pregnancy, the young man who impregnated her ran away, deserting her.

In retrospective images shown in Figure 3.33, Agnes overhears her parents negotiating a bride price for her marriage to an old man.

Figure 3.35

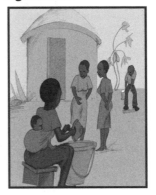

> *Mother:* He has offered two goats, a cow, a saucepan, and 50,000 shillings [Ugandan currency].
> *Father:* We cannot refuse him.

In Figure 3.34, bride price is given, and Agnes marries the old man as his third wife. The old man tells Agnes that his other wives will treat her well. Agnes joins her co-wives. As the third and youngest wife, the old man favors Agnes. In Figure 3.35, her co-wives are not happy.

> *First wife:* She thinks she is educated. She is only selfish. We will educate her.
> *Second wife:* Maybe the old man loves you . . . but we decide things.

These conversations reflect how a premarital pregnancy can catapult a young mother into a shamed life. The truth of this story is revealed in its dialogue.

I use language to reinforce social pressure and to show how cultural beliefs inspire vulnerability, as in an example in the story *Widow Inheritance*. In this story, when one brother marries his deceased brother's widow, he no longer pays attention to his first wife. His second wife gives birth to a baby boy, and everyone is happy except the first wife. When the baby boy dies, the second wife says to the first wife, "I know you have been doing witchcraft! It is you who did this!"

When a husband seems overly compliant with his wife's wishes and refuses the attentions of other women, his wife is sometimes accused of witchcraft, because it appears she has undue control over him. In this story, after the second brother dies, the third brother, Ogwal, refuses to marry the second brother's widow, and the widow, feeling insulted, tells Ogwal's wife, "Your husband has greatly insulted me by refusing me" (fig. 3.36). In the next image, the rejected widow says to Ogwal's youngest sister, "His wife has bewitched your brother. He has refused me. He brings shame on my family and me."

In this second image in Figure 3.36, market women are looking at Ogwal's wife saying, "Did you hear that this woman has bewitched her husband? He no longer has interest in other women. A very powerful love potion, indeed!"

It is likely that Ogwal's rejection of the widow would be interpreted in this way: Ogwal's wife has put something in his food or done something to him that caused him to make this decision. Witchcraft is a common explanatory device for unfavorable, and in particular sexual and health-related, phenomena. Since the advent of AIDS, witchcraft accusations have increased.

The story *Helen and Robert* shows how important the Ugandan family and community could be in reducing forced marital sex. While there are cultural prohibitions against having sex during menstruation, after childbirth, and when a woman is sick, men sometimes disregard these prohibitions, particularly when they are drunk (Cash 2011). Before Robert and Helen marry, the adults from their families meet to negotiate bride price, as shown in Figure 3.37.

Figure 3.36

Amut me Imung
Mon Too

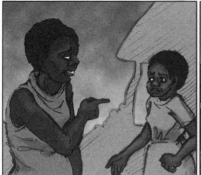
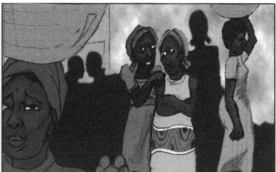

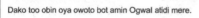

Dako too obin oya owoto bot amin Ogwal atidi mere.

Akullo: Omini be iloko ni ocamo yat oko ibot dako mere. Kong inen okwero laka oko. Man dong twon alano adit bota kede bot jo itur wa.

Naka jo ame tye icuk ocako kwoto Aceng oko. Kan ame obeo iye ducu inwongo jo tye akop ikome.

Mon ame tye icuk: Iwinyo ni dako ni oloo wi cware atek. Ogwal aman dong pe mito mon okene.
Mon okene icuk kunu: Dako ni omio cware yat atek ateteni. Ogwal pe twero gero dako okene. Okwero naka lako cii ominere aco en aye myero gwok otino atoo ca.

Figure 3.37

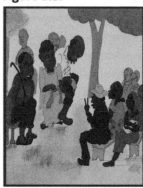

Figure 3.38

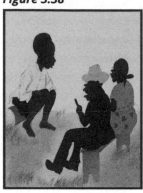

Figure 3.39

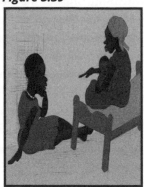

Then a parent, an uncle, or an aunt meets to talk to Helen and Robert separately about their marital obligations. In Figure 3.38, Robert's parents say, "Soon you will start a family. A man is the head of his household."

In Figure 3.39, Helen's aunt tells her, "Never turn your back on your husband in bed. When you disagree with him, keep quiet. Do not fight with him."

These words mirror the contradictions of forced marital sex, as Helen and Robert are told in essence that forced sex is acceptable since a wife should never refuse sex. On the other hand, forced sex is often due to shame-filled conflicts between married partners, which will surface as the story proceeds. In Figure 3.40, Robert's family welcomes Helen.

In Figure 3.41, Robert is drinking with his friends and discussing women. Robert asks why pregnant women often refuse sex with their husband.

One friend says, "When women are pregnant, sometimes they are rude."

Another friend says, "Yes, they don't want the husband around."

Helen says, "It's not good to play sex [a literal translation meaning to have sex] now that the baby is ready to come out" (fig. 3.42). Then Robert appears drunk at the door (fig. 3.43) and in the next images, he forces Helen to have sex (not shown). This is the under-story.

Figure 3.40

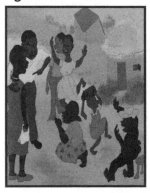

Figure 3.41

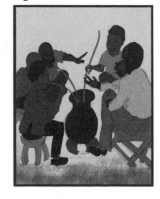

Figure 3.42

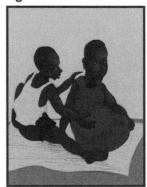

Figure 3.43

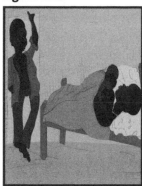

Figure 3.44

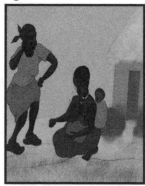

Figure 3.45

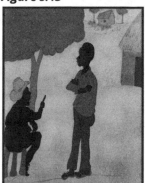

Helen tells her mother-in-law what Robert has done (fig. 3.44), and she says, "His father must speak to him." In subsequent images (not shown), Robert is angry at Helen for telling his mother, saying that sex is his decision. However, in Figure 3.45, Robert's father says, "Son, you must be patient while your wife is recovering."

Then the father talks to both: "Daughter, once you recover, you should not refuse your husband. Son, you must control yourself. Please respect each other" (fig. 3.46).

Figure 3.46

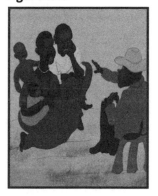

In the Ugandan story *Rumormongering*, neighbors intervene to try to stop domestic violence. The dialogue shows how Ayena (the husband) feels suspicious of Atala (his wife) because of the rumors he hears about her. The dialogue in Figure 3.47 reflects how others contrive to create conflicts between married partners. Ayena is talking to his male friends who tell him, "You must watch your wife. She is very friendly with a young trader." In the third image, the text reads, "Ayena worries. He looks at Atala. He is looking for signs."

In Figure 3.48, a man warns Ayena, "Observe your wife closely. Don't just listen to rumors." Ayena wants to play sex, but Atala says, "I am tired. . . . I worked too hard today . . . so I will sleep with the children." In the next image, Ayena is drinking with his friends and they say: "Reaching the bed . . . fight the vagina and let the vagina cry."

In the first panel in Figure 3.49, Ayena beats Atala. Ayena says, "You lie! Are you a prostitute who moves from place to place . . . as soon as my back is turned?"

Atala says, "No! No! You are wrong . . . it is you . . . it is you who is playing sex outside. It is you who is overlooking [to shame by ignoring or by not responding] me!"

In the second panel, the neighbors intervene: "Ayena! Ayena. . . . Stop this! Enough! This is not the way . . . not the way."

Figure 3.47

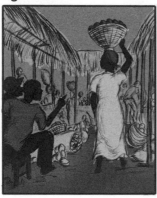 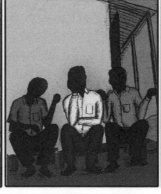 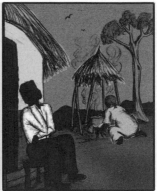

Awatere me acel: Gwok dako ni nono aber pien en ame ineno tye awot icuk nono, jo ducu nwongo tye amwonyo lao ikome dang nwongo tye amito yamo kede.

Awatere me aryo: Ayena, dako ni nono tye ona kede acat wiloro icuk kan ame ka pe ineno aber, awobi twero mayo dako ni oko.

Figure 3.48

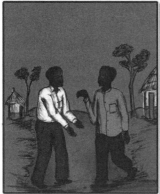 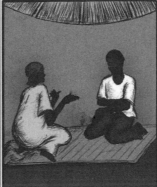 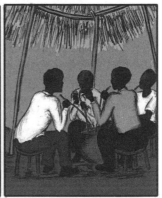

Awatere me adek: Kong inen dako ni nono kong idiro. Pe ibed winyo kop awobe wad wu pien kare okene kop ame gin okobi obedo kop goba.

Atala: An aol atek en ame ibedo yela nono ...tin amako ticogo atek cakere odiko naka otyeno. Ka ibedo yela atek, wek awot abut piny kede otino name aweki wi tanda.

Owote Ayena: Pe inii dako bed loyop wii pien pe en aye onyomi. Wot idony ikabutu ...teki okwero ni pe ibut kede, yab lweny ikom dako wang ame kome ame en tye awanyo kede nono dang okok.

And in the final panel of Figure 3.49, Atala reports Ayena to her parents, saying, "He falsely accused me. The man I talked to wants to marry [my] Sister"— meaning that the man Atala was talking to was trying to negotiate a marriage with Atala's sister. Atala says this to justify why she was talking to a man in public (the basis of the rumor that resulted in violence) though it is unclear whether Atala's justification is true or not.

— —

Thus, through character dialogue and imagery in the story *Rumormongering*, the reader hears and sees how violence caused by rumors escalates over time.

Figure 3.49

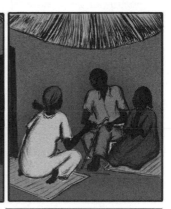
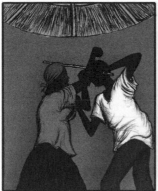
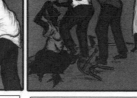

Ayena: Wek kobo goba pien amaki wun icoo moro tye ayamo kedi! Inito kobo ni yin ibedo malaya ame ilongo piny ikabedo ducu teki ka ineno koma orweny ipaco.

Atala: Pe amano...Pe amamo kadi acel! Wek kodi kop goba ame icako ikom jo nono gik oko tin! Yin aye myero bed ni itye iture...kopi nono nyutu ni yin aye itye imito mon ooko. Dok dang inaro butu ked gi bala gwogi ame tye atepo. Amito kobi tini ni pe iwir bal ame yin itimo iwia!

Jirani: Ayena! Ayena...wek lweny bedi! Ipwodo dako ni dang oromo! Dako pe olwenyo kede alwenya kadi otrino bal. Lweny pe kit ame opwonyo kede dako ka otimo bal. Tubere ka tye iot otyeko abedo.

Atala: Cwara obin onwonga atye akop kede awobi moro eka te dwogo paco ame yie tye awang ni an amito awobi naca. Aco awobi naca onwongo tye akoba ni emito nyomo amina atidi nu.

11.

From the Thai program, the story *Lamyai* describes the expectations a Thai family has of a daughter and the expectations she has of herself, leading to her unexpected, tragic end. *Lamyai* is about a young Thai woman who migrates from her rural village to the city of Chiang Mai to work in a garment factory. Her family plants a lamyai tree, the girl Lamyai's namesake, to mark the day she will leave and the day she will return. The tree in the story becomes a romantic metaphor of natural beauty, fruition, and rebirth.

The text in Figures 3.50 and 3.51 reads:

"You know what I would like to do with my 50 Baht ['Thai currency]?" Lamyai said with a mysterious tone. "I would like to buy a small lamyai tree and plant it in our front yard. Then every year when I come to visit, I will see how it has changed and grown. Like me! And when this tree is full grown . . . when its fruits are the most delicious, then I will come home to stay and never leave again." A

Figure 3.50

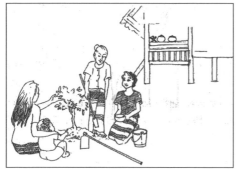

Figure 3.51

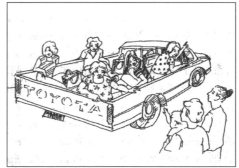

feeling of deep sadness enveloped their family as they planted the small tree that afternoon. The next morning Lamyai left for Chiang Mai.

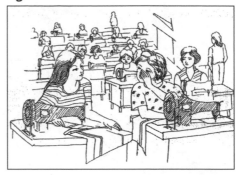

Figure 3.52

In the voices of the characters in this story, the reader hears the sadness of Lamyai's departure. Lamyai is a good child who is fulfilling the cultural obligations of the youngest daughter by working to support her family (fig. 3.52). This sets the stage for the emotional impact of Lamyai's return as a daughter with AIDS and subsequently as a daughter whose promise of return is in her death.

The voices that speak in the text are ultimately the readers' (Brooks 1984:304). Dialogue in interactions between characters sets the stage for conversations during the practice (Chapter 4, Step 5), when participants are asked to respond to a story crisis: *What could she have said? What could he have said? What could have been said differently or done in a different way to have prevented a crisis, a conflict, or a tragedy?*

Salient and Colorful Imagery

They reached out to their emotionally charged visions and tried to touch them, to hold them in place, perhaps on soft surfaces with their fingers. They were not inventing images. They were merely touching *what was already there.*

—*David Lewis-Williams,* The Mind in the Cave

I marvel at the power of belief that images evoke. Images as straightforward as a person dying of AIDS or a man beating his wife or a woman beating a child: "We saw the child being hit with a big pot, sleeping on a floor while everyone else was in a bed with beautiful sheets, where the child is walking barefoot to bring other children to school and doing all the work in the house like cooking, collecting sticks for the fire, fetching water and cleaning the house. Well . . . maybe we knew this before, but now we believe it." The difference between knowing and being aware is essential. Being aware connotes belief. An image invokes belief though the observer might have known about what the image is suggesting before he or she saw it. When I began working in HIV prevention, I realized that the people I worked with knew useful facts about this disease but were doing little to prevent it. Emotions cultivate belief though these emotions must be shared: "We see actions; we hear the story and what people are saying. Now we believe it!"

Text alone cannot achieve the strength and significance of a story that also has visual imagery. Because many participants in these programs are marginally or non-literate, it is important to create meaningful and relevant imagery so that people can tell the story. Some programs provided a printed book for each participant to take home. Therefore, it was essential that a participant with book in hand would be able to tell the story to his or her family or community independent of the text, if he or she could not read. In order to achieve this, the critical events are illustrated in separate frames. The illustrations define events in such a way that the participant can tell the story without reading it.

I work closely with artists so that images will convey the meaning of the text. To choose artists, I meet with them and read a story. After this reading, I ask the artists to create one image for the story. The artists are selected based on their ability to render an evocative image rather than because of their credentials or educational background. For example, art in Haiti is revered, and there are many rural, itinerant artists (who illustrate the walls of voodoo sanctuaries) with no formal art training or employment. Sometimes I show artists' images to local people to see how they respond, because I do not feel culturally equipped to evaluate local artists' work.

The process of working with artists is lengthy and collaborative, taking over two months of intensive work in some cases. Because I am a visual artist and educator, I have a sense of how visual representations can work together with text to achieve an educational result. On occasion I have found an image missing when I can no longer meet with the artist, for instance, when I have already returned home. In these cases I create the image using the style of the artist, but I have never redone or edited an artist's work.

In the process of illustrating a story, the artist first reads the story that she or he will be illustrating. I discuss the story with the artist, and then, as the story is being discussed, I sketch stick figure drawings to give the artist vague suggestions on how the image might be configured. I do not want to interfere with the artist's skills or creativity because I cannot foresee or imagine another artist's visual interpretations. Discussions and redrafting of images occur frequently until the final result. In one program, five artists with distinct styles discussed their drawings with each other, as they worked independently in the same room. In some projects, artists hand-painted their drawings. In others, I asked graphic artists to add color digitally to images created by artists in other countries.

In the Bangladeshi program, I did not use written text because the literacy of the participants where the program would be used was very low. The image in Figure 3.53 is from a story about a Bangladeshi girl and boy who fall in love. In this first series of images, a boy and girl meet, fall in love, dream about each other, continue to meet, and have sex.

The next series of images, shown in Figure 3.54, show what happens after an unmarried girl becomes pregnant. In the third panel she daydreams about marrying the boy. In the next panel, when the pregnant girl is collecting water, the other girls shame her. Adults talk to the boy and explain what will happen to him if he marries the pregnant girl (not shown). Finally, in the fifth panel in the figure, coerced by his parents, the boy is taken away to marry another girl.

Figure 3.53

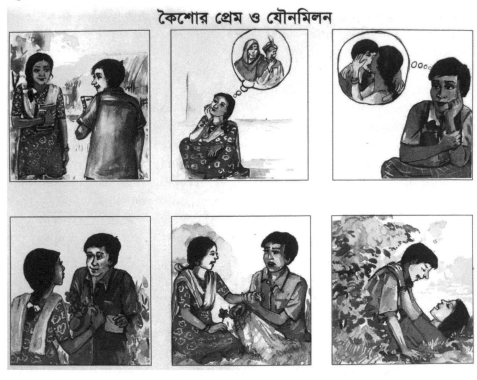

Figure 3.54

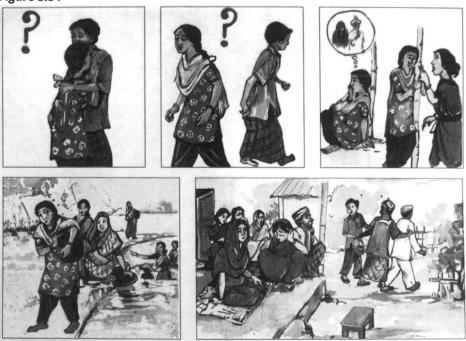

The point of this story was to encourage adults to talk to youth about premarital sex and the prevention of pregnancy. As more Bangladeshi boys and girls attend school, premarital pregnancies are an increasing problem for youth as well as parents and extended families.

Most programs include written text together with images. In the Haitian environmental program, the initial research revealed community conflicts over land rights, water usage, grazing animals, market trash, tree cutting, and many other issues. This program focused on how lack of community dialogue and collective action was increasing already severe environmental problems. Images reflect the severity of these conflicts. The first image in Figure 3.55 is from the story *Free Grazing*, which shows the consequences of not tying up animals. After untied animals devastate Malen's garden, she takes revenge by cutting off the head of her neighbor Enel's goat. This action initiates a cycle of revenge especially because this was not the goat that destroyed Malen's garden. Enel was going to use proceeds from the sale of his goat to support his children's education. The emotions of the characters are illustrated in their body language and the image of the dismembered goat. The images are dramatic and begin a story of how an irrational act of revenge led to further acts of retribution.

In the story *I Am in the Market . . . I Can Put My Trash Wherever I Want!*, from the same program, market women talk about dirt and dust in the market (fig. 3.56). Evelyn says they should go to the local leader but Mary Lourdes says, "Sometimes misery is ruling. We are obligated." Mary Lourdes secretly defecates behind the market cattle.

Later, her child is sick from eating unclean food, and Mary Lourdes sees the consequences of her actions when the market floods. The images in Figure 3.57 reflect a crowded market, uncovered food, and open debris, and after the flood, the visual suggestion that Mary Lourdes' feces polluted the market grounds. Each image reflects how disease can spread from lack of market cleanliness.

Figure 3.55
Elvaj Lib

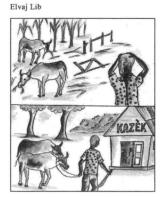
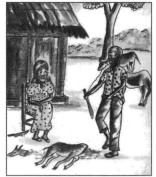
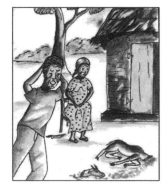

Figure 3.56

Se nan Mache a M Ye, M Ka Lage Fatra Kote M Vle!
Istwa Sekrè

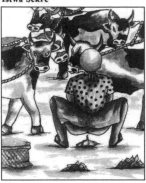
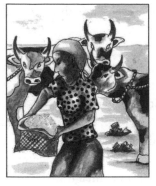
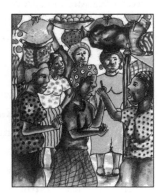

Figure 3.57

Se nan Mache a M Ye, M Ka Lage Fatra Kote M Vle!

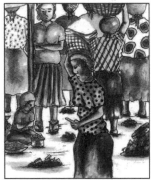
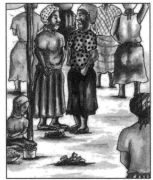
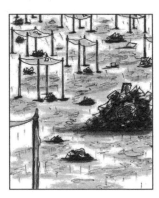

In another story in the Haitian environmental program, *Food for the Soil*, the images explain how Dadou and his wife prepare the soil correctly according to an agronomist's advice (fig. 3.58). The agronomist explains the negative consequences of burning soil.

Dadou and his friend, Wilson, both hear the agronomist's advice and publicly agree that it is not good to burn land, but later Dadou sees Wilson's fields burning (fig. 3.59). Wilson tells Dadou that a child playing with matches set his field alight. Wilson and Dadou both know it is faster and less work to burn one's fields than to turn over the soil or to add organic matter.

Later in this story, Wilson is suspicious of Dadou. He thinks that Dadou has practiced voodoo on Wilson's land so that his land did not produce while Dadou's did (fig. 3.60). The visual lessons of the agronomist, images of land burning, the characters' pensive examination of their fields, the comparison of the different yields from Dadou's and Wilson's fields, and the suspicious look of Wilson reinforce the story text.

Figure 3.58

Manje pou Tè a

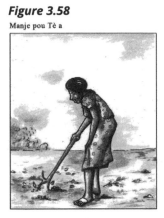
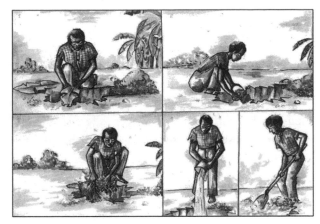

Figure 3.59

Manje pou Tè a

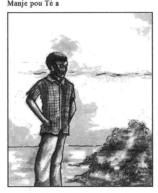
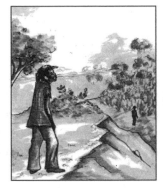
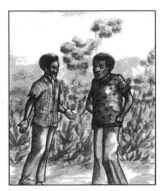

Figure 3.60

Manje pou Tè a

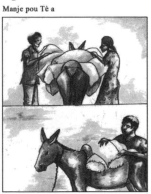
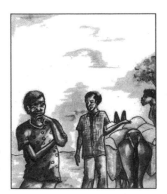
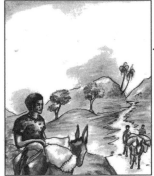

Excerpts from *Is This What She Is For?*

I will show how the text, imagery, and structure work together in two complete stories from the Haitian children's rights program. The first story, *Is This What She Is For?*, begins with an image of Josette at age fourteen working as a servant (fig. 3.61). The next image is a retrospective one of when Josette was five years old and a man told her that she must become a servant because her mother had died and her father can no longer take care of her. In the third image, Josette is working as a servant and socializing with other servant girls who tell her that if a boy likes her, he will give her a new scarf: "If you have a boyfriend, he will buy you one too."

In the next series of images, shown in Figure 3.62, Josette's social inferiority is illustrated. Josette is a caregiver to boys who are her age and who live in the same household where she works. While the boys sleep on a bed, Josette sleeps on the floor. Josette bathes the boys and carries their books to school, though she is not allowed to attend.

In the third image, Manno, the youngest boy in the household, befriends Josette, which foreshadows her demise.

Figure 3.61

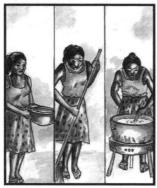
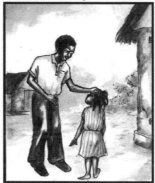
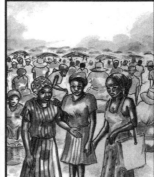

Figure 3.62

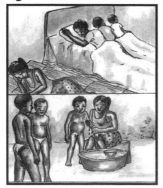
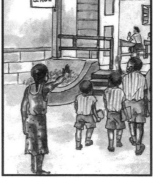
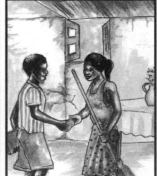

The next series of images, in Figure 3.63, are the under-story. Manno gives Josette a scarf telling her, "Don't tell anyone . . . they will be jealous. They will think I'm trying to buy your affection." Then they make love and afterwards Manno tells Josette, "No one has to know about our love. . . ." When Manno gives Josette a scarf, she believes he loves her as she loves him, reminding the readers of what Josette's girlfriends said to her earlier in the story.

In the images in Figure 3.64, Josette's friends remark about Josette's new scarf, teasing her that she must have a boyfriend though she denies it: "You are smiling these days . . . we think you have a boyfriend. Where did you get the new scarf?" But Josette will keep her promise. She does not reveal her love for Manno.

In the next under-story, Manno's older brother Jacque calls Josette to his room saying "Josette! Can you help me?" Then Jacque rapes Josette.

Following this, Josette sees Manno with another girl. Josette's friend tells her, "Oh, that Manno . . . he is quite the lady's man" (fig. 3.65).Then the last image shows that Josette is now pregnant. She overhears Manno and Jacque talking about her. The descriptive text reads "A few months later Josette is showing she is pregnant." Josette hears Jacque talking to Manno (fig. 3.66). Josette does not know what to do. The brothers are trying to decide how to get rid of Josette so they do

Figure 3.63

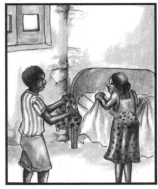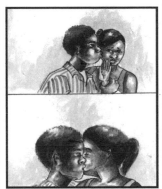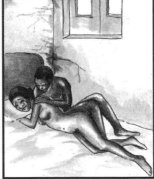

Figure 3.64

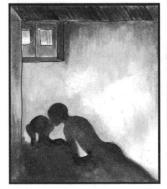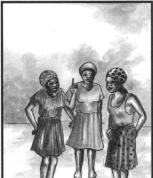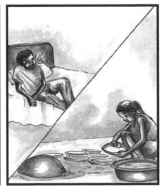

Figure 3.65   *Figure 3.66*

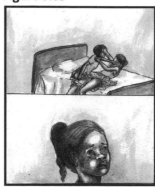 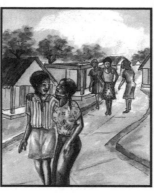 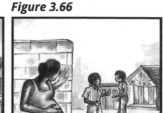

not have to take responsibility for her pregnancy. The dialogue between Manno and Jacque reiterates the story title:

> *Jacque:* Josette is starting to show she is pregnant. I had her once. . . . Isn't this what she is here for? Mother will beat me if she finds out. Better send her away!
> *Manno:* It could be anyone. She must pack her bags . . . these girls from the rural areas are whores anyway.

As part of community narrative practice, which I will discuss in the Chapter 4, "The Pedagogy," after program participants read the story, they discuss this un-resolved ending.

Excerpts from *I Took an Animal from the Road, So I Will Return It to the Road*

In this second story from the Haitian children's rights program, *I Took an Animal from the Road, So I Will Return It to the Road*, the first image in Figure 3.67 shows a child in servitude carrying a calabash of water. Often children in servitude are dressed badly or their hair is unkempt, as this image suggests. Here, women from

Figure 3.67

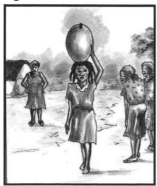 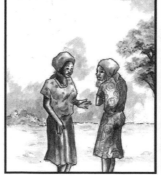 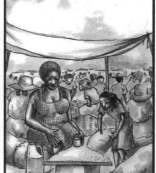

the neighborhood are whispering about the treatment of this child, Ester saying: "Mimose treats her like a dog," and "Mimose is without patience . . . she knows she can mistreat this poor child. The child has no voice." In the third frame Ester is working for her caregiver, Mimose, in the market. The image contrasts Mimose, who looks fat and strong, to Ester, who looks skinny, weak, and overworked.

The next three images, in Figure 3.68, show Ester sleeping on the floor, while everyone else sleeps in a bed. The family is still sleeping when Ester gets up very early to fetch water, which is a common obligation of children who live in servitude. As it is not uncommon for children in servitude to be teased, while Ester is carrying water, boys tease her saying, "Hey, you . . . ugly girl . . . come over to me! Come here . . . suck my dick! You think you are superior . . . flies won't land on you!" Ester fights back and breaks the calabash filled with water.

The images in Figure 3.69 reveal the under-story. Mimose beats Ester for breaking the calabash saying, "You can't play when you fetch water. I will teach you!" I learned from research respondents (former child servants) that often they were made to do work beyond their physical capabilities—like carrying heavy water jugs.

In Figure 3.70, Ester carries water in a large bucket, but she drops the bucket and skins her knee. Mimose hits Ester with a shoe, saying, "You are a stupid, ugly

Figure 3.68

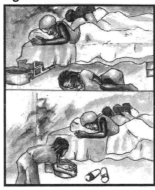 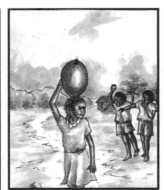 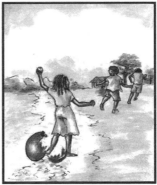

Figure 3.69   **Figure 3.70**

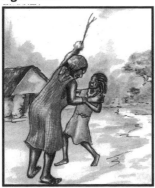 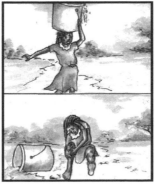 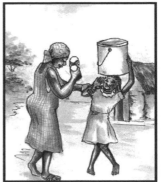

Figure 3.71

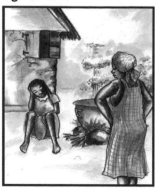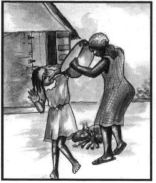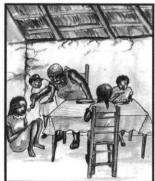

girl! You don't learn . . . you are so ignorant!" A caregiver or a parent might hit a child with a shoe, their hand, or a green stick. These images evoke strong emotions from the audience. They see how a child in servitude is being mistreated as the mistress beats her for each infraction. Because of the images, participants experience the plight of Ester as witnesses because the story itself is a testimonial.

Following this, Ester falls asleep while the food is cooking, not an uncommon occurrence if a child is overworked. The food burns. Again the under-story reveals that Mimose not only hits Ester with a pot, but also refuses to give her food. In Figure 3.71, Ester is sitting on the floor while the family is sitting at a table eating.

Mimose says, "You stupid, wasteful girl! You can cry blood but I am not giving you food today!" One of the mistress's children pleads with her mother to give Ester food but Mimose refuses (fig 3.72). When the daughter says, "You have hardened your heart to this little girl," Mimose counters with "I took an animal from the road, so I can put it back in the road," echoing the story title.

Then the child's father is called to talk about the behavior of his daughter. The father's manner, standing hunched over with hat in hand, shows his obsequiousness toward Mimose (fig. 3.73). He says, "Madame, I am most obligated to you." The father talks to Ester about her behavior, telling Ester that he cannot take her home. In the final image, in Figure 3.74, the child Ester is working again. The same women who appeared at the beginning of the story whispering about the mistreatment of Ester comment again about her abuse with varying points of view:

> **Woman One:** If she stays in that house, that woman will kill her for sure. She gives the girl work that is too much for her years. Should we not do something?
>
> **Woman Two:** These little girls . . . they develop. All Mimose put into her will be wasted. In a few years she will be pregnant and run away or Mimose will have to put her in the street. These mountain people have no education. Mimose is doing what she can.

Figure 3.72   *Figure 3.73*   *Figure 3.74*

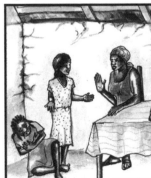
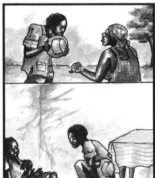
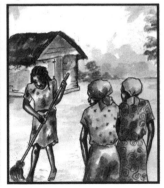

The last image and dialogue merge with the pedagogical questions for program participants: What do you think about what these women are saying? Why didn't these women do anything even though they knew this child was being mistreated? When you see a child who is being mistreated, what do you say, what do you do? What could you do to help this child and prevent further abuse?

Many participants will have witnessed similar incidents in their community. Perhaps they felt empathy, but they did nothing. The reappearance of the women at the end of the story is a visual and textual reminder to the audience of what it means to do and say nothing. The narrative intention is to invoke awareness and shame in the audience (see Chapter 4).

Contextualization creates the recognizably *real*. In order to contextualize a story, I select and develop verbal and visual symbols learned from the ethnographic data. Think of the plot as the frame of a story and of the character dialogue and imagery as the contextual outer layers that add cultural and emotional meanings. I spend a great deal of time and thought trying to get it right, meaning trying to capture actual words, phrases, dialogue, and effective imagery. Together, dialogue and images create a mirror in which participants can reflect on themselves and others. Unless there is emotional resonance in the story, it will neither be believable nor transformative. Consider this:

> Suppose that the world either was impervious to our emotions, or instantly and utterly capitulated before them. Suppose, for instance, that, whenever we loved someone, our love was never returned, not out of indifference or because love had been pledged elsewhere, but because the thought of such reciprocity never occurred to the person. Or suppose that, whenever we were angry, the object of our anger dropped down dead. Our emotions either totally determined the lives of others, or made no impact on them whatsoever. Furthermore suppose that this was, not only how the world was, but how, in our phantasies, we represented it. Our emotions would, I suspect, die of the lack of interaction, of the lack of narrative. (Wollheim 1999:224)

4 | The Pedagogy

You are hearing the story . . . getting these emotions and these reactions, and you hear someone say something . . . what she went through . . . and you felt you were the only one. You think "I am not crazy for responding the way I did." This is what happens. This is a powerful thing. Silence, what flowers in the African American community, is really driving up this epidemic.

—a facilitator from the African American Program, 2002

A shared narrative is what matters. Reason does not turn the trick.

—Lev Vygotsky

A Brief Overview of Step 5: Practice

This is a practice of public engagement. The force for transformation is not in the composite narrative per se as a non-dynamic entity, but in the structured practice of dialogue with, and in the presence of, others. The constant presence of, as well as the interactions with and affirmations from, others is central as people begin to think about and/or to tell their own stories. A transformed community narrative comes into being only from people's interpretative discourse about the story. In this way, the composite narratives become a means of transforming the *self in relation to and with others*.

Phases of Community Narrative Practice

1. Discussing a Seminal Image (Distancing the Self)

Everyone sits in a circle. The monitor asks a timid person for an opinion. Everyone participates. Participants are giving their opinions about what they know. I think when people participate like this, with this sharing, they hold on to it. For example, when I ask, "What do you see in the image?" a participant might say, "I see a woman standing up with a pot in her hand." But when the teacher just describes it, it bypasses the listener; they forget it. When participants comment about the images, when they enter into this kind of dialogue, it can serve them in society.

Figure 4.1

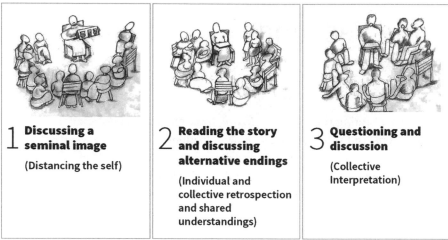

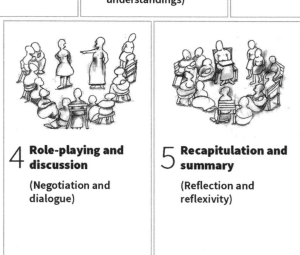

At the beginning of every session, the facilitator asks the group to respect each other's opinions and confidentialities. In the first activity, the participants look at a seminal image from the story without text. Participants respond to questions about the image. The facilitator asks the participants the following questions:

- What do you see in this picture?
- How do you think the characters in this picture feel?
- How do you feel when you look at this picture?
- Do you see any problems?

There are no correct answers to these questions. Participants answer freely without comment or criticism on what they or anyone else has said. This seminal image will appear again within the context of the story as it is read. Participants will then recognize this image and think back to how their interpretations fit with the actual meaning of the image in the context of the story.

This introductory activity involves all participants at the outset of a session. Communities from which participants are drawn have long-standing hierarchies. This activity democratizes the learning process because it allows for engagement without evaluation, encouraging the voices of all participants. This is critical because it sets the stage for the rest of the practice.

Figure 4.2

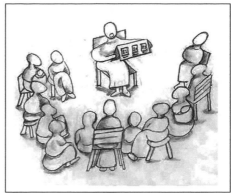

This first activity distances and engages the self. The seminal image causes detachment or separation: "Only people are capable of this act of 'separation' in order to find their place in the world and enter in a critical way into their own reality" (Freire 1973:105). This objectification of the image leads to a separation of the viewer from the image—a distance strengthened by the analytical questions the facilitator asks. This enhances critical thinking and awareness. This objectification creates a belief in the truth of the image, perhaps an *elusive truth*, but nonetheless the certainty that we are here in a common experience, which will be reinforced when this image reappears in the context of the story.

The reappearance of the seminal image achieves an aha moment as a participant thinks, "Now I understand." The seminal image at first is really a flash-forward (though participants might not see it as such) to an event in the story. During the reading of the story, the image reappears, and each participant's thoughts flash back to its first appearance before the story was read. At its reappearance, separate understandings of the image crystallize into a collective interpretation. This heightens confidence as participants experience a unified awareness of the narrative's significance.

The seminal image is central to the theme of each story. Here are a few examples:

In the Latino program, from the story *Victoria's Secret*, about transsexuality, shame, and HIV risk, I chose a seminal image that shows Victor's father exchanging a doll for a truck when he sees his child Victor playing with a doll (fig. 4.3). This picture will later appear in the story when Victor's father sees him playing with a doll and chastises him for it.

Figure 4.3

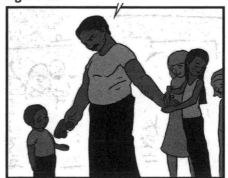

From the story *Who Is This Man I Thought I Loved?* about domestic violence, I chose an image where the young woman, Claudia, is seeking help from her parents. Later this image will appear

Figure 4.4

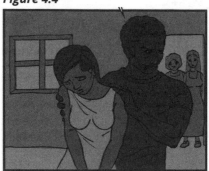

Figure 4.5

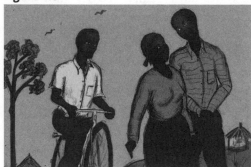

in the story when Claudia's parents encourage her to return home with her husband, Raul, because of the shame Claudia might bring to the family if she leaves him. Here her husband is taking her home as Claudia's parents look on (fig. 4.4).

In the Uganda program, from the story *Rumormongering*, I chose an image showing a woman happily talking to a man while another disgruntled man is riding behind them on a bicycle (fig. 4.5). Later this picture will identify the various characters and how this event signaled shame, accusations, and eventually violence.

From the story *Girl Child*, I chose an image of a woman and a man holding a baby while others appear to be looking on (fig. 4.6). For rural Ugandans there is no indication in this picture that the baby is a girl, but there are contrasting facial expressions between the people holding the baby in the foreground and the people in the background.

In the story *Widow Inheritance*, I chose an image of a man in the foreground who is clearly sick and two people in the background who appear to be comforting each other (fig. 4.7). Later on this picture will appear in the story when an older brother is dying of AIDS while his younger brother comforts the older brother's wife whom he stands to inherit upon his older brother's death.

Figure 4.6

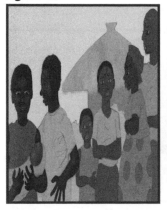

Figure 4.7

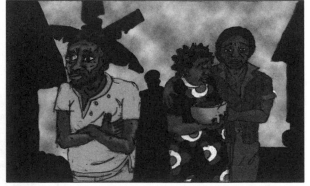

Figure 4.8

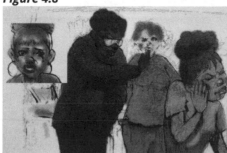

Figure 4.9

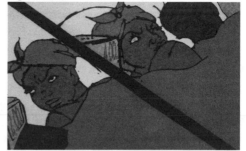

In the African American program, from the story *Mama You Don't See Me* about child molestation, I chose an image of a teenager being slapped across the face by an older woman (fig. 4.8). I inserted a small picture of the same girl as a crying child, apparently looking on. Later on this picture will appear in the story when a teenager is slapped because she is openly hostile to her mother, though her hostility reflects the concealed truth of the under-story.

From the story *If I Revealed Myself, Would I Be Cast Off?*, about a married man who is on the down-low, I chose an image of a woman looking at a clock at two a.m. when her husband is not in bed with her and then again at four a.m. when he is (fig. 4.9). In the story this picture will appear later on after an under-story where her husband has been at a party having unprotected sex with a man.

In summary, this first activity invites the interest and involvement of participants. They are immediately introduced to the program's methodological intent and questioned. I want to actively engage participation from the beginning of each session and stay with this purpose throughout. Each participant should feel from the outset that he or she is a part of the learning group and his or her participation is essential.

Creating separation between participants and the narrative at the beginning intentionally detaches participants, creating *narrative objectification*. Exhibiting an image that is distanced from the self, critically questioned, and collectively acknowledged builds the truth of the narrative.

2. Reading the Story and Discussing Alternative Endings (Individual and Collective Retrospection and Shared Understandings)

After participants leave, when they are faced with a problem similar to what was heard and seen in the story, their memory will go back to the story . . . it will stay longer with them when they come to a similar situation. "This happened to me."

After the seminal picture is discussed, the facilitator reads the story (fig. 4.10). Whether participants are literate, marginally literate, or non-literate, they follow the text by reading, listening, and/or looking at the images. In some contexts, the books were incorporated into a literacy program. Participants read along with the facilitators or took turns reading a story out loud, sometimes with the facilitators' assistance. Because some had gone to school many years before and often for only a few years, over time their literacy had declined. The books helped these participants improve their literacy.

Figure 4.10

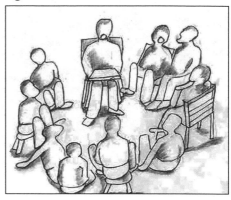

There are questions throughout the story. Sometimes the facilitator asks these questions, but usually participants want to hear the story without interruption. During the reading, the facilitator will often say "under-story," signaling its appearance before it is read.

Listening to the story is a retrospective experience, invoking memories of past events and feelings. Aspects of the story will resonate with some people's personal experiences. Others might feel connected to the story by knowing the experiences of others such as family, friends, or neighbors. In some instances, some participants call out "under-story," predicting its appearance before it is read. Frequently the participants, because they are actively involved in the story, make comments, laugh, and express anger, sadness, or embarrassment while the story is being read.

Most stories do not have an ending. Where the story stops, the facilitator asks participants, "How would you end this story?" Or in some cases, "What do you think is going to happen next?' Often story characters are in the midst of a critical decision that the participants must complete. For example from the Latino program, in the story *Who Is This Man I Thought I Loved?*, Claudia finally calls the police when Raul begins to physically abuse her. When the police ask Claudia if she wants to press charges, she hesitates. Participants discuss Claudia's options and the consequences of each.

Sometimes when the story stops, story characters are in the midst of asking themselves or another character a question, which the participants then answer. At the end of the child molestation story *Mama You Don't See Me*, the main character, Dee, asks Angel how she can protect her own daughter (protection that Dee's mother had failed to provide for Dee) from a fate similar to her own. At the end of the story *Helen and Robert*, about forced marital sex, Helen wonders whether Robert will force her to have sex if she refuses in the future, and if so, what should she do? The participants share ideas in response to this question, which also brings up their varying points of view.

When a story ends in narrative practice (usually when a decision or action needs to be made), there is no narrative resolution. Peter Brooks comments about interpreting narrative plot: "If the motor of narrative is desire, determinants of meaning lie at the end, and narrative desire is ultimately, inexorably, desire for the end" (1984:52). What happens in the narrative when the desire for resolution is stymied by its absence? The no-end is asking for extended narrative possibilities, which will, according to Walter Benjamin *close the sentence as a signifying totality* (quoted in Brooks 1984:22). Narrative closure, in this practice, is not the storyteller's or the writer's or the individual participant's alone, rather it is derived from the audience. In this there is reflexivity that shifts between the composite narrative and participants' retrospections about related events in their own pasts. Participants publicly discuss and share interpretations of possible and alternate narrative endings and with this, they reinterpret possibilities within their own lives.

As participants discuss alternative endings, they also engage in shared understandings. Sometimes participants share private experiences. Sharing personal stories creates the dynamic of testimonials and witnesses, and this validates the truth of the composite narrative. Testimonials bring the private plights of individual participants to light. Personal experiences of participants give credibility to the story and, at the same time, participants who have not experienced the problems of story characters serve as witnesses. Witnessing a testimonial and seeing oneself in others affirms the commonality of shame.

This practice builds solidarity among participants and the feeling "we are in this together." However, being in this together does not mean the participants are victims. This sentiment would be counterproductive because it would ignore the ways in which pathways to shame can also be pathways to pride. Sources of pride suggest narrative possibilities. Listening to recognizable personal experiences transfers themes of a composite narrative to a recounted reality and to realizable strategies. If these shared interpretations ignored examples of past agency, this practice's dialogic intent would run aground.

3. Questioning and Discussion (Collective Interpretation)

People learn to accept the ideas of others even if what a participant says is not totally correct. For example, if someone says something and the facilitator keeps asking questions to the other participants, soliciting more interpretations, the person will say, 'Oh, I thought I was right but now I see things another way.' This approach finds agreement between people with respect. With this method participants' minds are more open.

Figure 4.11

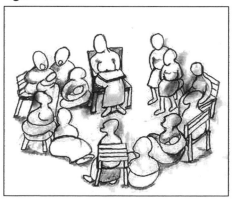

At the end of each story there are suggested questions for discussion (fig. 4.11). Participants share their interpretations as the facilitator asks these questions. Because the list of questions is long, facilitators choose those questions most pertinent to participant interests and time.

Discussion questions focus on relational problems and dialogic crises in the story. Because the learning sessions emphasize conversation, the discussion questions in turn focus on what could have been said and how. The facilitator might ask participants to give advice to story characters. Some questions ask how the characters might have talked or acted differently such as, "What would you say or do in this situation?"

Questions also focus on gender-based and age-related issues, such as different expectations for men and women and how these affect behavior, attitudes, risks, and interactions. For example, in the stories about forced marital sex, discussion questions focus on poor communication and a gendered perspective of shame and how this leads to violence. Or, in the stories about youth, discussion questions focus on poor communication between youth and adults and how this puts youth at risk. In stories about interactions between women and men, questions focus on how gender expectations and roles play a part in their conflicts.

These discussions encourage participants to learn from each other and think critically and dialogically. Most participants have knowledge of the issues beforehand, but have never discussed them in a public forum. Or, for some, particularly for women and youth, they might have heard discussions of the issues but did not feel confident to speak. Discussion encourages shared interpretations, focusing on how and in what ways conversations between characters led to conflict. This builds participant self-confidence, because it gives participants practice in speaking about the issues.

Individual participants answer questions posed by the facilitator. But instead of a rhetorical approach, the facilitator encourages dialogue between participants by not only asking questions directly to a participant, but by also asking fellow participants to comment on what others have said. This type of questioning encourages dialogue between participants and moves the control of the discussion away from the facilitator and into the group. This is another strategy geared toward creating solidarity and consensus.

4. Role-Playing and Discussion (Negotiation and Dialogue)

To be honest, I couldn't express myself before. Now I can. If someone is not acting well, anyone will go to replace that person. This made us ready to help one another. Sometimes you keep repeating it until you get it right. This helped me. Those who were watching . . . they would tell me 'well done!' This made me feel proud and motivated. We felt united. When you go home, things stick in your memory because of the role-play. You don't forget it fast.

Role-play is a public-spirited, dramatized means of exploring various types of engagement—confrontation, negotiation, dialogue, reconciliation, and resolution—around a point of conflict or tension between story characters (fig. 4.12). Like the questions for discussion, at the end of each story there is also a list of possible role-play topics.

Ordinarily the actors have three chances in each role-play to change the nature of their interactions. When the actors have reached an impasse, the facilitator suggests they try again. As an example, from the story *Girl Child*, the facilitator and participants decide to dramatize a conversation between Adong and Adur where they are discussing Adur's desire to take a second wife because Adong has failed to give birth to a boy. In the first chance: Adong

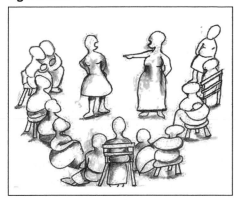

Figure 4.12

and Adur are in conflict; Adong does not want Adur to take a second wife, but Adur is angry because Adong has not given birth to a boy. In the second chance: Adong and Adur try to negotiate or get past shame, blame, and anger. In the third chance: Adong and Adur try to reach a resolution. Unfortunately, in some role-plays the conflict will not be resolved to each party's satisfaction. However, this is one of the goals of role-play—to critically reflect on how conflicts are resolved though sometimes not equitably and/or to everyone's liking. In conflict, Adong's voice is heard; however, in the resolution it might be silenced.

In these role-plays there is lack of separation between the spectators and the actors, for at any time they can change places. The drama or role-play occurs in the center of a ring formed by the other participants (fig. 4.13). At any point in the role-play, an observer in the ring can become a performer or actor. If someone wants to speak, but he or she is not an actor, that person taps an actor on the shoulder. When this happens, the actor and observer change places. The actor goes back into the circle and the observer stays in the center as the actor. This gives anyone a chance to play a role and add comments during a role-play. Changing actors offers different interpretations and varying points of view. Also this is a means of building self-confidence and group solidarity.

A role-play with the help of reflective judgment can give rise to a moral analysis. Ordinarily in a drama or role-play, the audience shares emotions, reflection, and a critical community (Lara 2007). However, reflective judgment from the audience's perspective alone is imbalanced when the audience remains the outsider looking in. Reflective judgment, according to Lara, consists of linking action to judgment: "This first happens when the spectator or reader issues a judgment about what is happening in the representation, where she

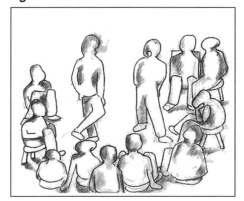

Figure 4.13

considers the idea of a spectator who sees action with an impartial detachment. The second moment occurs when spectators engage in understanding action, to pursue new paths to transform themselves" (2007:44).

In narrative practice, when spectators and actors spontaneously switch roles, they are experiencing reflective judgment not only in a spectator's objective view or in an actor's subjective one, but in their merger. The role exchanges of spectator with actor achieve a more profound and balanced moral perspective in a combined experience of the actions themselves and in the external judgment of those actions. In this, for the participant, reflective judgment is experienced within a recognition, awareness, and understanding of the other. This is particularly significant to gender- and age-related conflicts where seeing a situation through the eyes of the other can achieve more equitable compromises.

The role-plays are politically charged in that the drama gives people the chance to reenact and publicly change dynamics of power and powerlessness. In the role-plays, shame is actualized as actors and the audience reenact shame-filled conflicts—how they arise, how they evolve, and sometimes how they are resolved. Actors select different strategies to approach and talk about a shameful problem. They name shame.

By publicly acting out shame-filled paradoxes, the drama ironically acknowledges the consequences of silence. This demystification of shame, in its public reliving, bends the public narrative. The shame of any one person who has personally experienced this crisis is not in question. However, the public narrative that has laid claim to silence, that has given rise to private suffering, is. Who among the audience (participants and passers-by) does not know this hidden text?

The role-play is a chance for people to practice how to listen, what to say, and how to say it. Unlike a typical drama, the role-play involves participants in constant engagement since they are audience and spectator, and, as both, they are asked to listen, respond, and think critically throughout.

In one program, where mediation was a central need of participants, I asked each actor to paraphrase what the other actor was saying in the second round of a role-play performance. Thus the role-play became an exercise in highly focused listening and interpreting as well as in speaking. This exercise was put to good use later on when participants applied the skills they had learned in the role-plays to help them resolve community-wide conflicts.

Participants who were non-literate consistently commented that the role-plays really helped them remember the story. They said that after they left the learning sessions, "the story stayed with us" because of the role-play.

In order to learn more, after the role play the participants discuss what happened. The facilitator engages the actors and the audience in discussion of these questions:

- How did you feel as an actor?
- How would you have liked to have changed your role but circumstance prevented you?
- As an actor, what did you learn by participating in this role-play?
- How did you feel as an observer or in the audience watching the role-play?
- How do you think the actors felt in a particular scene? How do you know this?
- What would have been said or handled differently within the context of this role-play and/or in a real life situation in your family or community?
- What have you learned from this role-play?

As actors and as spectators, participants consider their feelings about the role-play conversations and actions; they become more acutely aware of both the emotional and the bodily feelings that the story characters they are portraying might have experienced. So they might think and discuss: "How did I feel as the actor, Adur, when against Adong's wishes, I was telling her I am going to take a second wife?" Or, "How did I feel as a spectator listening to the conflict between Adur and Adong?" Reflecting on the experience of being an actor and/or a spectator is central to this practice.

By observing and then discussing the role-play, participants learn to think critically about role-play interactions, which will aid in their confidence to speak once they leave the program. While text-as-performance in a role-play evokes an emotional, cathartic response (Denzin 1997), among actors and audience there must be a critical response as well.

People are entertained and emotionally engaged as they watch and perform in the role-plays. People who were not in the program sometimes came to watch the role-plays. Many spoke about how much they appreciated being in the audience even though they were not regular participants in the program. Also, in the beginning of some programs, ill-founded rumors prevented people from joining the program (see the section titled "People Talk about Challenges" in Chapter 5). The role-plays helped dispel these rumors.

Following the role-play and the role-play discussion, the facilitator reads corresponding health, children's rights, or environmental information depending on the focus of the program. This part of the session extends what participants learned from the narrative to learning about related factual information. After this information is read to the participants, they ask questions and talk about it.

6. Recapitulation and Summary (Reflection and Reflexivity)

The methods influenced my life. When someone is talking, I listen closely to what that person is saying . . . and the more I show that person I'm learning from him, he will give me more information and he will be ready to receive information from me.

Each session ends with a discussion about paradoxes and problems brought up during the session (fig. 4.14). The group is called upon to summarize the session, and then, in conclusion, the facilitator encourages participants to take what they have learned from the program to events and problems outside the session. The facilitator asks participants to share the stories with family, friends, and neighbors as she or he emphasizes that they, the participants, take the title of some of the programs,

Figure 4.14

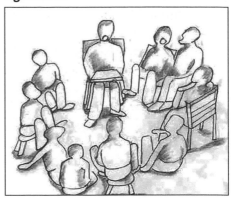

Education Is a Conversation, to heart. Ideally participants have a book in hand that will help them tell or show the stories to others. Finally, at the very end, as at the beginning, the facilitator requests that the participants fulfill their commitment to confidentiality for any personal information divulged during the session.

Deconstructing Narrative Practice

I was on my way to the marketplace, and I saw this woman hitting a child with a big stick. I said, "Come on lady, you are not supposed to hit a child like that anymore." The woman said, "Oh she did too much to me." I said, "That's not the best way. That child will be replacing you, and when the time comes, she will be treating her children the same way you treated her." So I gave that child, who was about six years old, to a neighbor, and I said to the neighbor, "Please wait until she calms down before you give that child back to her. Where I come from, people don't hit children like that anymore."

This practice engages people in a process of individual reflection, collective retrospection, interpretation, dialogue, enactment, and reflexivity. Narratives set the stage for participant engagement. Participants see images within a story that call up a lived past and an anticipated future. The narrative pedagogical process intensively engages each person in a social process, building on the notion that "the subjective is always social and the social, subjective" (Kleinman and Fitz-Henry 2007:64).

In experiencing a story that visually and linguistically represents the known or familiar, the audience is at the same time distanced from it. Participants see and hear how power and powerlessness are deconstructed within story content and context. The audience experiences the demystification of vulnerability, but they are not subject to feelings of vulnerability because they stand outside of it while they observe characters and listen to the story. This observed experience causes reflection. One might then reflect or think critically back to private incidents without revealing one's story publicly.

The stories exemplify the relational struggles in a public deconstruction and reconstruction of the dialectics of inequities in human interactions. Story characters' shame transfers to participants' retrospections. Through narrative paradox, participants reinterpret lived expectations and frustrated desire. As story characters transact and renegotiate their lives, participants reflectively do the same.

Roland Barthes writes about the text of pleasure and the text of bliss:

> Text of pleasure: the text that contents, fills, grants euphoria; the text that comes from culture but does not break with it, is linked to a comfortable practice of reading. Text of bliss: the text that imposes a state of loss, the text that discomforts (perhaps to the point of a certain boredom), unsettles the reader's historical, cultural, psychological assumptions, the consistency of his tastes, values, memories, brings to a crisis his relation with language. (1975:14)

The texts used in narrative practice are texts of bliss. The participant hears, sees, and/or reads the paradoxes within and between the top- and under-stories. This praxis moves learners through different modes of experience. The language and imagery of the story draws the audience into the emotional experiences of characters. But there is also a separation, a break with cultural submersion, however subtle. In that there is a state of loss.

There is the observed experience—the state of bliss is the state of loss of one's own or another's powerlessness. In other words, a state of concealed loss is replaced by a publicly powerful recognized powerlessness. There is a *real* loss of shame, which is a loss of a past self because the hidden text is exposed. The revelation of loss is in the collective and public naming of narrative disappearance, an unacknowledged story of private plight within everyone's sight. To maintain a state of *narrative disappearance*, forbidden acts must be submerged. In a state of *narrative appearance*, they are no longer submerged. This state is felt within newly configured legitimatized shame, in a revised public narrative. And herein lies the power of this narrative practice: it can collectively transform public narratives and because of this, enable people to change their lives and help others.

As the story is read, the listener reflects. Each participant asks him or herself, "Am I not looking at myself?" or, "Isn't this me that I am observing?" or, "Don't I know these things already?" As previously discussed, the audience feels a sense of shame (self-loss) in that which was supposed to be hidden (his or her failure in the eyes of the other). The audience experiences a state of bliss—released from this loss of hidden shame—and is, at the same time, asked to respond morally and generously to others.

In this practice, to be the onlooker to another's demise (which is also a testament to one's own) evolves into a redefined collective authority. The emergence of this collective authority marks the beginning of public narrative change. This authority of experience in renegotiating shame is transformative because it is a reflexive experience that achieves authenticity out of dialogue and collective awareness. This experience is neither exclusively derived from the composite narrative nor from the pedagogical process but from the merger of the two.

Transformative community narrative practice is a collective route to people's deeply felt emotions and interactions. Narratives provide routes into memory. A collective response provides possibilities for narrative transformation: "Ways of telling and ways of conceptualizing that go with them become so habitual that they finally become recipes for structuring experience itself, for laying down routes to memory, for not only guiding the life narrative up to the present but directing it into the future" (Bruner 2004:708).

The pedagogical process engages people in collective interpretations. Moving from silence to conversation, from conflict to resolution (or lack thereof), from invalidation to credibility, there is public confirmation of shared sentiments and beliefs. The audience is witness to the top- and the under-story, to the dialectic tensions and transactions between the texts and in explications of failure and of agency. There are irritations that need soothing, fragmentations that need totality, shameful feelings that need reconciliation.

From the beginning of each session to its end, narrative practice is a process of constant, continuous, overlapping, and evolving engagement with others. The key is dialogue. Interpretation is only made possible in dialogue. From conversations with each other to taking on different roles, in practicing what to say and how to say it, people learn from each other. They reflect and discuss possibilities for change. They listen to story characters' experiences that mirror their own, and talk about commonalities. They give testimonials, or, as witnesses, they listen, and together they interpret and reinterpret. And by the end of each session, they have arrived at various ways they might change their own and others' vulnerabilities. In all of these processes and outcomes, there is the emergence of new forms of community solidarity. Together they have arrived at new feelings of confidence. The participants finally have discovered ways to constructively talk about things they could not talk about before.

5 | Evaluation

I told my friends that this program really changes people—even if you are someone who does not want to be changed you will. Once you negotiate and learn to talk in a good way with each other, fighting will stop. I loved this program so much. Anyone can find something that reflects his own life. I would join it again.

—*a young man from the Uganda Program, 2012*

Flaws and Possibilities

When I walk in rural areas in developing countries and ask people, "Is the next village very far," people will invariably answer, "No, it's very close—just over there." Then they point as though my destination is just over the next hill. A day or two later I'm still walking. Anyone I ask will say the same thing. I don't believe people are lying in the sense of trying to confuse, hurt, or play a joke on me. Rather they don't want to disappoint me. They're telling me what they think I want to hear. At times, this kind of graciousness is a challenging obstacle to finding out a program's 'real' impact.

There are unforeseen challenges when I use traditional evaluation approaches with people who are not literate or marginally so. Evaluators tend to be outsiders in that they are more educated, wealthier, and worldlier than respondents, and thus have a higher status than them. To please the evaluator, the respondent believes she or he must put on a good face. This means telling the evaluator what the respondent thinks the evaluator wants to hear.

Feelings of appreciation for a program are not necessarily tied to truth telling. When people are asked a question where a truthful answer might be critical of narrative practice, they might withhold criticism. This might have to do with a participant's relationship to a supporting organization, which might be helping him or her outside the program. It is unlikely anyone will be critical if he or she believes it will hurt this relationship or the organization itself.

Moreover in some contexts evaluation is used as a means to punish or chastise, not as a means for improvement. I once observed this when foreign consultants innocently recorded honest evaluations, thinking that these evaluations would help improve worker performance. Instead this led to employee dismissals.

Quantitative surveys are particularly difficult to administer for a variety of reasons. Because of participants' low literacy, it would be very difficult, if not impossible, for them to read questions and fill out answer sheets. I provide an answer sheet to each participant, and questions are read aloud. Together, participants tick a blank on the answer sheet after each question is read.

In a read-aloud group evaluation, older respondents have problems understanding and remembering questions. Most have never filled out an answer sheet and this presents new challenges.

Not sharing answers is a foreign idea. I feel odd asking respondents to hide their answers or to sit far apart when they have just participated in a program that emphasized sharing, open communication, and collaboration.

I try to get over some of these hurdles by conducting an evaluation survey in small groups or in large groups with supervisors continuously circulating to make sure people are not sharing answers. However, there are always surprises. In one place, people called out an answer and then everyone ticked it in unison. In another, out of frustration, evaluators asked people to answer a question by raising their hands. Everyone waited until the first person raised a hand and then immediately followed suit. When asked to close their eyes, people squinted to be able to give the same answers as their friends.

I use a variety of evaluation methods and within these look for means of verification. Ordinarily I create two types of instruments, a quantitative pre- and post-survey to test for measurable change, and a qualitative unstructured instrument (similar in style to the ethnographic research guide), to assess change that is difficult to quantify.

In my opinion, evaluation methodologies should complement the methodological goals of narrative practice. Because the goal of a program is to influence conversation, I believe the form and substance of a quantitative instrument must be able to measure conversation change. In one program, I had respondents answer questions about taped conversations I played for them. In another, I wrote about a crisis with different choices of character conversations. I asked respondents to select the most appropriate conversation for a specified outcome.

Invariably in qualitative evaluation interviews, I discover that participants applied what they had learned in ways I had not predicted. If one does not understand how people might apply what they have learned, how does one formulate a quantitative question to elicit information about this? Qualitative evaluation is better for uncovering the unexpected.

Quantitative evaluation in general is more suited to cognitive change and changes in specific actions, while qualitative evaluation is better suited to actual changes in conversations within interactions. Qualitative evaluation lends itself to the subtleties of emotive and nuanced change that is critical to understanding the impact of narrative practice.

Means of Verification

Qualitative evaluation interviews might provide anecdotal rather than *real* evidence. Therefore, I analyze qualitative data in the same way I analyze ethnographic research data, by looking for patterns and repetitions and by avoiding anomalies. Evaluators are trained in the same methods as ethnographic researchers. For example, extreme statements, such as, "I don't have sex anymore unless I use a condom" or "I've stopped drinking alcohol" are red flags, which suggest further questioning is needed.

A fruitful means of verification is to interview children, youth, neighbors, partners, and family members of program participants—people who were not in the program but have had contact with or know a participant. Children are reliable respondents. In one incident, the participant emphatically told me that she no longer hits her children. But when I interviewed her son and asked him if his mother hits him, he said, "Yes, she hits me but no longer with a pot or big stick. Now she only uses a little stick."

Another child respondent verified what her mother (a participant) had reported. She talked about a child in servitude living in her household:

> Since mother has been in the program, she doesn't hit us anymore, because the monitor of the program said she must not hit children. She used to hit us with a bat, whip, and *frete* [green stick]. Now when the little girl [*restavek*] takes her things, she doesn't hit her. The little girl has improved. They talk to her. There is more harmony in our house. Now they tell us why we shouldn't do things.

People Talk about Changes

For qualitative evaluation, I am interested in how the participants' lives are different because of the program and how they interpret those differences. I am also interested in why the program might not have affected them, and if it did not, what might have prevented them from achieving the changes they desired. Ordinarily I select three different categories of respondents for evaluation interviews: the program participants; people outside the program who did not participate directly in the program such as partners, family, children, neighbors, and friends of the participant; the staff who implemented the program including facilitators and supervisors. For each group of respondents, I write a separate semi-structured interview guide. I gear the questions to reflect gender- and age-specific interests. From the program participants, I am interested in what they learned; what changes the program brought to their lives; what obstacles they faced; who they talked to about what they learned; why they chose that person to talk to; what they said to the person; and what the person said in response. I want to understand the circumstances that caused a participant to use the skills he or she gained from the program. I want to know about changes in knowledge and practices (including risky behavior); in feelings about the self and others; and in relations and interactions. I also want to know what activities they liked and why, and what narratives they remember and why.

For spouses, children, relatives, friends, and neighbors of participants, I ask them to explain how a participant's behavior changed since he or she was in the program; whether the participant talked to her or him about the program and what she or he said; whether the program had an impact on that person's relationship with the participant; why the respondent thinks the participant talked to him or her; if this had any effect on that person's life. If the answer is yes, I want to know how things changed. I also want to know what they heard about the program and why they did not join.

For facilitators, I am interested in what changes they saw in participants from the beginning to the end of the program. I am interested in what learning activities participants liked and why, and what obstacles the facilitators faced in managing the sessions and how they coped with these.

Facilitators were asked to take regular attendance and keep a record of what happened during each session's activities. I want to know if attendance or time management was a problem and why; what participants disagreed about and why; about surprises—things the facilitator had not expected; and about the impact of the program on the facilitator's life. The facilitators are generally living in the same communities and facing the same issues as participants. In one instance, a facilitator learned she was HIV positive during the program when her husband, who had hidden his status from his wife, became deathly ill.

Over the years, I have read hundreds of evaluation interviews from the eight different programs. Ordinarily the evaluators and I interview approximately one third to one half of participants, a sample of program outsiders (like children or spouses or neighbors), most of the facilitators, and some staff of the supporting organizations. Usually the facilitators set up the venue and the interview appointments with participants or others. Each interview takes from one to two hours to complete. The following is a brief overview of what I have learned about narrative practice from these interviews.

Changes in Knowledge and Practices

Respondents are asked specific questions about what they learned in the program about HIV and AIDS, condoms, sexual and reproductive health, children's rights, or the environment, depending on the content of the program. For example, in the sexual and reproductive health programs, there is factual information about HIV and AIDS, STIs, male circumcision, RTIs, condoms, ARVs, puberty, fertility, and sexual and domestic violence. As a consequence of the program, most took an HIV test, some a second or third time and some a first: "I realized I was so stupid and ashamed of myself in that I didn't mind about my life. I got my blood tested, found out my AIDS status, and got examined. I felt this program gave me courage to know my health status."

Though ARVs are available, people still fear contracting HIV and AIDS. Program participants chose different strategies to alleviate their fears of transmission:

> The training changed my life because now I take care of my life. Before our relationship was the worst but since the training I don't hate him so much. I got the

courage to tell my husband to go for a blood test. I learned about HIV. When he refused, I decided to refuse sex with him. This training changed my life because I don't depend on my husband as before. I do my own business. I feel a lot of freedom because he no longer shouts at me like before when I was a beggar to him.

In evaluations of many HIV/AIDS prevention programs, the professed frequency of condom use is often questionable because these are not congruent with rates of transmission. Besides the discomfort and reduction of pleasure associated with condoms, people feel shame in regards to condom use with a husband, wife, or steady partner because it signifies loss of trust. Some people say that because of the program they now use condoms regularly or all the time saying, "I won't have sex with my husband [or wife] unless we use condoms." So ordinarily I do not believe these extreme pronouncements of change without further evidence.

On the other hand, in the HIV and AIDS programs, a common outcome was that women not only talked about condoms, but also gave their husband a condom when he traveled away from home. Some reported: "I told my husband—I'm going to ask you a favor, if you ever have an affair, I want you to use protection . . . if you don't do it, I want you to use protection with me. You don't have to tell me."

A wife's open, straightforward acknowledgement of her husband's risk and the subsequent risk to herself and their family was a milestone of prevention in some quarters (see Chapter 8). Men influenced by the program reported using condoms with a casual partner, but not with their wives. However, consistency of condom use was difficult to determine. Nonetheless, when a woman's spouse was in the program, her persistent questions and suggestions were reminders that likely had an impact on a partner's condom use with others.

Some participants knew the people in their community who were HIV positive and had refused ARVs. They talked to them: "I realized people fear to go to the hospital . . . then when it is very bad, they are taken but they don't respond to the medication because they are too sick. They just die. I know how to approach them now. Since the program, I have talked to ten people because I saw how they were declining. Now I have knowledge I can share with them."

Often participants chose people like themselves to talk to about HIV prevention or ARV treatment: "I don't think about brothers-in-laws to inherit me . . . since my husband died, I stay alone. I talked to Acan because she's having the same problems as me. She's a widow . . . she's infected. She never wanted to join ARVs but I ended up convincing her to. The training helped me because it gave me courage. I'm encouraging her to be strong-hearted like me."

An acknowledged risk factor for HIV infection for African American women is from a male partner who is on the down-low. A few women, to the surprise of other participants, openly testified having a male sexual partner on the down-low put them at risk for HIV infection: "She told us she was positive. It hurt me to see her hurt like that . . . she cried. She couldn't figure out where she got it from because the only person she was having sex with was her husband."

This is a shameful topic that participants began to address in more direct ways than they had before:

> Recently, he got in contact with me. . . . I told him about the AIDS program. It's a high-risk situation for men in prison. I would like to know what kind of activities he's dealing with. I let him know he needs to be tested. It is not a win or lose situation with me. I let him know I know certain things now . . . it's not going to be like it was before. I talked to him about homosexuality . . . his sexual preferences . . . his booty busting.

For the first time, husbands and wives began to talk openly about forced marital sex, a common source of partner conflict and a cause of HIV transmission in some places:

> I would ask him, "Why do you always force me to have sex with you? Tell me!" And he would say, "Whenever I want it, it means I want it!" Then I would ask him why he wants to do it when the children are still awake. He would become quiet. The biggest problem in our house was forced sex when he was drunk. Now if we want to have sex, we have it, but if one person doesn't, we leave that person to rest. It's because of the program. Now we respect our children and ourselves.

Men and women in separate groups had different conversations about forced marital sex. In women's groups, they discussed how to react—whether resistance makes things worse and whether forced sex is against their rights. Some said they did not know they had a right as a woman to refuse sex.

This young man explained the impact on the program on him and his friends:

> I chose to talk to my friends about forced martial sex and HIV and AIDS because it is the core of life here. Sincerely, women used to see men here as rapists . . . many men did this under the influence of alcohol. Many took my advice because they know I am a true friend who tells them things that many people are silent of. I tell them imprisonment and HIV are waiting for you when you rape. I used to think of raping girls with a bad group of friends. Before this training, we did not speak of women's right to make sexual decisions. No one would talk about it except the clan but this only happened when there was a serious fight.

Alcohol instigates many conflicts between married partners. Some of these conflicts provoke public embarrassment:

> My husband came home drunk . . . honestly . . . asking me for sex and food on the road before he reached home. When he got home, I am ready to fight him over the bad words he has used in public. Now I open the door and give him food but I am silent. In the morning I talk to him about his abuse. My husband didn't

bother to chat with me but he found a book and started reading it. That day he started chatting and then he came to the meetings and sat silently watching the training. I'm happy . . . really . . . there's been change.

While participants did not suggest that alcohol drinking should be stopped because it was a source of camaraderie and relaxation for men, most felt it was the extent of drinking that was problematic. Loss of household income or children's school fees, infidelity, and forced marital sex are common problems related to alcohol drinking:

> She fought back but she lost a tooth. She went home and vowed never to return. Then one day she talked to me about forced sex when her husband is drunk. He would treat her like an animal during sex—not respecting the child next to them. I felt she needed this program. I showed her the story of *Helen and Robert* but the husband complained that I was only supporting his wife. So I counseled both of them. I told him to respect his wife and listen to her, and I told his wife not to deny her husband sex so often. It's my pleasure to say that the husband thanked me for restoring their marriage.

One learning group was made up of men who met regularly to drink alcohol. These men met to chat about politics, women, or just to relax. In one men's drinking group, eighteen men out of twenty-five admitted to forcing their wives to have sex. When I returned, after the program ended, I asked the men the same question and three men told me that they were trying to stop, but as of yet, were unsuccessful.

Both men and women are unhappy about forced sex because it causes shame, hatred, and violence between them (Cash 2011). As this woman explained, "He used to scare me . . . whenever he was drunk, he would force me into sex. I felt my whole body was in pain. I don't know how he felt, but I used to hate him. When I tried to talk to him, he said, 'You just want to get rid of me and get another man.'" Before the program, women and men did not know how to constructively address forced marital sex. Many told me the program helped them do this.

An unexpected finding was that some participants perceived that the absence of child spacing was a cause of forced marital sex since forced marital sex often occurs when women refuse sex while recovering from childbirth. One husband agreed to child spacing after reading a story about forced marital sex: "When my child was twelve months, I had another pregnancy. My husband did not accept child spacing. Then he said, 'This must be known by many' after he saw the story of *Helen and Robert*. 'We have to practice child spacing to come out of this situation like the couple in this story.'"

Often a participant used one story as an example to talk with a person who reminded her or him of a character in the story. This became a means of talking to a partner about an uncomfortable subject such as infidelity and loss of income:

I shared the story of the fisherman with my husband because he is a womanizer. I said, "Don't be like the fisherman. If you don't stop, we will be separated . . . I will go to my place and remain there." After mentioning divorce, the man said, "These people who advise you to go to your home are misleading you. But I'll stop doing those bad things." We now dig together. Now he is upright and he reminds me to go to the program. Because I have knowledge from the program now, if he gets another woman, I'm not going to hide.

Along with the story *Girl Child*, I included a brief visual description using XX (mother) and XY (father) symbols to show how each parent contributes one chromosome to the child, but that it is the chromosome from the father that determines whether the child is a boy (XY) or a girl (XX). One husband explained how this affected him:

We talked that I should not chase my wife, but I should see a way of helping her and taking full responsibility for my family. This story helped me understand that the man determines the sex of the children and not the woman. Personally, it was a problem because the first, second, and third children were all girls. I thought my wife had reproductive problems . . . she is no longer blamed as she was before.

A husband, together with co-wives, the extended family, and the community, sometimes hound an infertile woman or a woman who gives birth to only female babies. Here a woman talked about how the information in the program affected her:

He brought a co-wife and he left me with my children. He wouldn't support me and saw me as a fool. The co-wife didn't produce and they separated. Women have XX and men have XY—so it is not necessary to blame the woman . . . that's how the story resolved issues about giving birth to baby girls. My husband used to really complain, "Why are you only producing girl children and not boys?" He was thinking of chasing me away, but after he got the training, he realized that I was not willingly producing girls. Before people gossiped that I don't respect my husband. Now I tell them, "These books are really helping . . . that's why you see change in my house." These days we don't quarrel.

Changes in Emotional Expression

When people get angry and lose control, they sometimes cause emotional or physical damage to each other. Narrative practice influenced how people expressed anger:

She didn't respect me and she tried to undermine me. It stopped. Earlier on when she was angry at me, she didn't talk to me, and I beat her up. But nowadays she calms down and tells me the whole problem—how it has happened. When she tells me about my mistakes, I apologize. I didn't apologize before. I didn't believe it was good to lower myself to a woman. Now I have knowledge, and I know sometimes it's a good thing to do.

Others spoke about how narrative practice helped them handle problems by being less reactive: "The program advocates for peaceful solutions. Now if I am annoyed, I cool down and then handle the problem. That helps me have control over my emotions."

Rumormongering was cause for intense emotional reactions if not physical violence in many locales: "I've learned it's really good not to react to something about you . . . it could be a rumor . . . someone hates you. She says so-and-so is talking about you. At times I might be fighting about nothing. I learned to investigate first. When people backbite, it's so painful, but it's not good to fight."

Some spoke about how men, in particular, did not know how to express their emotions constructively and the program helped them do this. A facilitator talked about the impact of narrative practice on men in a day treatment center:

It was awesome! Each participant kept coming back because they were learning more stuff in a personal way. At first they were learning something they didn't know they were learning . . . a lot of them don't know how to communicate their emotions. Then they realized they just helped a character . . . someone in a situation they could relate to without getting angry . . . without cursing . . . without using [crack cocaine or heroin] behind it. They realized, I can do it! They are less fearful of talking about personal issues now. The motivation came from within themselves. The program pulled it out of them. Unlike other AIDS programs, this one empowered the individual to be able to talk about delicate issues.

Changes in Oneself

Perhaps one of the most noticeable changes in all programs was the extent to which participants expressed newfound confidence and courage. One young man stated:

This program made me feel I'm the one who can determine the life I want to live . . . whether positive or negative. Others can talk but if the decision is not from me to change, change can never come to my life. This program made me value myself as someone very important to my community and my family. I can help others to change from fighting to negotiation.

Across all programs, participants used these words to describe personal changes saying I am . . . *more aware, more alert, not embarrassed anymore, not shy, confident, secure, knowledgeable, well informed, more comfortable because I know a lot now*; and that a program . . . *helped me take action; gave me light; changed something inside of me, taught me how to value myself . . . how to appreciate myself*;

and *life is better for me now because of this program*. Some compared narrative practice to other programs with similar topics: "I feel comfortable cause other programs made me feel sad, but this one gave me a feeling of power, of strength. It was very positive."

Many commented on how a program relieved stress or how they benefited from the sheer entertainment and fun they had in the groups:

> Because of this training, I started socializing with people. I learned I don't have to sit alone and worry. I came to the group and discussed problems like mine. Widows still want to play sex; some drink. If you had a bad life like mine, you are used to worrying. So I learned to see the good and stop this habit of worrying. I used to think I can't manage to be a widow. The training helped me cope with life as a widow.

Participants talked about how they had learned to give up grudges. They asked for forgiveness: "If my wife wrongs me now, she always asks for forgiveness and I, myself, when I wrong her, I ask her for forgiveness."

The program for some relieved past shame while for others the stories caused shame. In this case, the woman had been a participant but her husband had not: "I no longer feel shame but my husband feels shame about things he used to do . . . shame if he thinks about the past."

Like this woman, many no longer felt shame about things they had been ashamed of before. Many said they felt pride in talking about something they had not talked about before:

> My happiness is from the courage I got to talk to my children about sex. I learned how to talk to children rather than to shout at them. I felt I needed to begin with my own children rather than starting from outside. I wanted to keep them safe . . . they all got tested for HIV and they are all negative. I have a last born who would not listen . . . she was disobedient. But now I'm happy because she listens to my advice. This program gave me the boldness to sit with my daughters and tell them, "If any of you has a friend, then go for a blood test first" and to my sons I said, "All of you are big enough and if you are tempted to have sex, please use a condom." Now my children are open to me about their secrets.

They reported talking with a spouse, or with a family member reiterating this phrase: "I am able to talk about issues related to sex without fear or shame." This lessening of shame extended from private conversations to public forums:

> Before the program, I used to fear talking about sex and saying vagina or penis. But I learned that talking directly and calling things the way they are makes people understand better. So this encouraged me. I no longer feel ashamed. I

can speak in public without fear . . . I talked about condom use in a community meeting when a man accused his wife of cheating on him because she wanted him to use condoms with her.

In many responses I heard people explain why they no longer felt ashamed about themselves. One woman said, "The program had made me feel better about myself. Before people would ignore me because I have no education. But this program has given me the confidence to speak out what I couldn't have said before. And people really respect me compared to before the program."

In most of the projects, the program participants were either not literate or marginally literate. Even though some had attended a few years of school, there was nothing available to read. So in time, their literacy declined. Participants felt proud to have the books and read them (even if this only meant holding a book and telling a story by explaining the pictures). Educated people had warned me that books were too foreign and of little value to rural people. I did not find this to be true. For one thing, the books contain many pictures. For another, being educated is a sign that one is somebody (see Chapter 8). Having a book increased a non-literate parent's credibility with his or her children who were often in school and knew how to read. Neighbors and the community at large saw a participant with book in hand as someone who was receiving something important: "People wondered how an unlearned person could cover six books . . . this made those who used to laugh at me respect me. I learned that I can learn so much in groups. I used to ignore any gathering . . . but this program has given me confidence to speak out."

The books also contributed to narrative credibility because they were beautiful to look at. Many commented on the truth of the images. Credibility is critical to a program that confronts cultural sensitivities. In this regard, *the medium is the message* is relevant in literate and non-literate communities alike.

Changes in Skills

Changes in emotional expression were related to the acquisition of specific communication skills. Participants were proud of the confidence they gained in being able to talk with a spouse, a child, family, or neighbors: "The stories helped me because they taught me how to mediate and negotiate to end violence and to even support the people in my neighborhood who are experiencing violence. Before I would just act. Now I know how to be a good listener. That can really solve problems."

Like this respondent, many spoke at length about how they had learned to listen to their children and control their anger when children misbehaved. Many had said they had stopped hitting their children with damaging objects and instead were only using a small green stick. Because of this, they explained there was harmony in their families. "Our children," they said, "are happier."

A participant, acting as a mediator, tried to bring conflictive parties together in order to get them to negotiate:

Last Wednesday, the wife to my brother-in-law had a grudge over money. The wife would blame him, and he would blame her. As I was walking by, I found them fighting—really physically fighting. I calmed them down and asked the cause. So when they told me, I started to mediate, but the wife was so resistant, . . . she would not listen to her husband or me. The wife had caused the problem. But I talked to the husband and said, "Do you know this problem will continue? So just forgive one another." I ended up calming the situation down. I learned so many things from this program . . . like many negotiation skills.

Changes in Conversations and Actions

With Partners

Conversations between partners improved, particularly if a participant took the books home. Sometimes partners who were formerly going to divorce reconciled.

Since I got this program, I decided to stay with him . . . my husband changed. . . . Whenever I come back from the training, he asked me, "What are the topics you talked about?" He wanted me to forgive him for all the wrong things he had been doing. We tested our blood. We were all negative. Now he doesn't sleep out, though it is not really easy to know how men behave. Now he comes back early. I see a connection . . . if it wasn't for this program, there wouldn't be any change.

I noticed that if a man attended a program and his wife did not attend, the effect on their relationship was more direct compared with couples where only the wife attended. This respondent was not in the program but her spouse was: "One time after a session, he came home and did what he never did before and he said, 'Everything that we do has to be from the consent of both of us.' He himself actually said that to me! I believe that it's this program that changed him."

Women participants sometimes had problems influencing a reluctant partner. When a husband was resistant, women enlisted the help of family members. Sometimes children shamed an adult by showing that person the books:

My husband is someone who is really hard with me and with the children. A lot of bad things come out of his mouth. I told him the story of Jerbon, and ever since, he doesn't do that anymore. Before my husband used to hit me a lot and made me feel really, really bad. I showed the books to my children, and they went to their father and said, "Look! Look at this stuff!" It made my husband really sad, and now he's not hitting me anymore.

Many women participants could not read. Having the books in hand, a wife could show them to her husband so he could read the stories himself: "I learned that he was having extramarital affairs . . . he would go sell the produce I had worked to produce. What he has been learning made him change. He's always reading the stories especially the one about this man who had too many women. This story touched him so much."

Not surprisingly, noticeable change occurred when both spouses were in a program (though usually not in the same learning group):

> He used to scare me. Whenever he was drunk, he would force me into sex. I felt my whole body was in pain. I used to hate him. When I talked to him, he'd say, "You want to find another man." Now when we want to have sex, we negotiate. He's able to listen to me. He reduced his drinking. It's because he's hearing the stories and seeing the pictures. He even told me, "I was doing something very bad."

In this example the husband and one of his wives was in the program. The husband complained that the co-wife who was in the program had changed, but he lamented that the one who was not in the program had not:

> If you compare the two—the one who is in the program listens. Our discussions are fruitful . . . it's easy to discuss things with her but with the other one it's not. The one in the program is more respectful of me . . . the other one is still rude. My wish is to change the other one to be like this one who was in the program.

Violence is often instigated out of the shame a man feels when his wife undermines him. Men reported that the program had taught their wives not to get angry but to listen and negotiate. Men said things like, "I feel this program has instilled discipline and respect for me." And women said things like, "When I share with him, he pays attention and responds positively compared to before; since the program, we sit and discuss, which never happened before."

Many participants said that the program changed spousal interactions regarding household decision-making: "When I get money, I plan with my wife for the education of my children. This is a change for me. I joined the group. Then my wife joined. I felt touched."

The words *touched*, *heartfelt*, or *moved* came up quite frequently in the evaluation interviews when people described the emotional impact of the stories.

WITH CHILDREN AND YOUTH

Ordinarily, youth do not receive adequate sexual health education in schools or from adults outside of schools. One participant used the books to teach youth in her community about sex. Once young people found out that a community member had this information, they sought her out, and she met with them privately. In another program, a younger brother commented, "My brother showed me the books because there are certain things I did not know. The elders don't tell you anything. This helped my life."

Participants talked with their children about condoms, sexual and reproductive health, delaying sex, and staying in school, amongst other things. Most participants said that they had never before talked to their children about sex. A combination of cultural prohibitions, lack of confidence, and not knowing what to say or how to say it prevented adults from doing this. Regardless of locale, sexual health education was rarely offered in schools, and when it was, youth felt inhibited to ask questions because of the possibility of being laughed at if they did.

Across all the programs whether parents were educated or not, they wanted to talk with their children, but they did not know how. When incarcerated participants' children visited them, they used this chance to talk: "This program gave me the courage to talk to him. When I saw him on Sunday I asked him if he was still protecting himself. I told him I got a lot of useful information about AIDS. He had the courage to tell me everything that's going on with him."

Information about genital hygiene, specifically how women and men should wash, was unknown by participants, and they shared this information with their partners and children. "The program helped us teach our children to avoid early sex, to go for an HIV test before sex and marriage, and how to take care of the hygiene, like how girls should bathe from front to back, which we did not know before—even my wife did not know this."

Participants said that overcoming this challenge improved their relationships with their children. Some said their children were happier, freer, and friendlier to them. This facilitator who was a community leader living in an IDP camp explained how his relationship with his daughters improved:

> I told my daughters, "You know you shouldn't fear each other. There are certain things that if I don't tell you, you might not know them . . . certain body changes like you might have started your menstruation but you don't know what it is . . . so from today onward things happen like this." Then I showed them the books and I told them, "It's not easy for you, but for me . . . it's okay . . . don't fear me now." They are closer to me now. When they went back to school, they asked me for sanitary pads.

Participants who had failed to converse with their children wished they had had this program before. Most parents had no formal education so sometimes their children who were attending school did not respect their parents' views:

> I was able to talk to my children about the program. I have a daughter. When she reached Grade 7, she got pregnant and that really created enemies between the parents of that boy and me. I ended up giving that girl to them and they deserted her. I have a young girl in Grade 6. . . . I showed her the books. The one who gave birth said, "I wish these books had come earlier. I would not have gotten pregnant, but you were not advising me like you advise my sister." Now I talk to

her freely. Now she respects me. Before she would ignore me or say I was backward . . . that I didn't know the modern world.

Women are often blamed for a daughter's early pregnancy because the mother
was supposed to prevent this from happening. Therefore, older women participants
whose children were adults used the books and information to teach youth in
their communities about sexual and reproductive health. In one setting a group of
women participants went to schools to read the stories to youth.

Children spoke as well about the pride they felt in being able to talk to a parent:
"My mother and I talked about the stories, and I showed her how I read. So I
learned if you have sex, you get pregnant. It's me who wouldn't talk to my mother
about this. I felt too shy to talk to her, but now we talk."

One young man spoke about the situation of youth and the importance of
talking with them about HIV, sex, and other things that are not normally talked
about. He even went to a school to talk to children there:

> We fear talking about sex . . . being young people it's hard to talk about these
> things because elders will say you are very disrespectful. They'll say you are a
> spoiled child. I realize now that talking about sex is not bad. Most of us got
> messed up because our parents didn't talk to us about sex. HIV is a very big chal-
> lenge. If we don't talk, then our community will be finished. I have the courage
> now to talk in schools though the students laugh, but they understand the points
> I'm making. I don't shy away now.

Many children were orphaned due to the war in Northern Uganda. They lived
within extended families, and often they were not treated as well as the children of
those families:

> I'm always sincere and I don't lie. I share the rightful things I've learned from
> these books and I talk with others in the program to find out if what I share is ac-
> curate. To my surprise, being in this program made people trust and respect me so
> much. I am an orphan. I was not taken care of. I didn't have any one guiding me.
> Even my husband appreciates the changes in me . . . like I no longer bark at him.

Participants reported that because of the program they stopped segregating orphans from their own children, as this woman explained: "Those who died trusted
you to take care of these orphans. I think the stories about orphans really touched
me. It gave people deep thinking that orphans should not be used as a tool to gain
wealth or as child labor. That moved me a lot."

A newly married woman inherited orphans from her husband's brothers, one
who had died in the war and the other who had died of AIDS. She had had difficulties caring for the orphans she had inherited:

This program enabled me to hold hearts and treat these orphans as my children. In the past, I used to ignore them and take them as other people's children, and I didn't want them to bother me with anything. These days I feel like I am a real woman in my house. Thanks to this program, they are really free with me. When I ask them to do something, they do it without any complaints and when they want something, they ask me, "Mother, I want this." If there is money, I give it.

I went to the elementary school to talk with some orphans. One orphan was living with the respondent above, and I wanted to verify what she had said. This is what the child told me:

Now she is quite friendly. She is not harsh when she talks to us. Now there is no segregation [meaning differences in treatment of orphans compared to the children of that household] and we live together as one family. She taught us about hygiene. I think she did the right thing. Before, talking to her alone was a big problem. She would shout, . . . sometimes cane us. She no longer canes us. I think that this program is meant for adults to learn to treat orphans better.

With Family, Friends, Neighbors, and the Community

Many participants lived in extended households. When participants took the books home, this opened up conversations amongst family members and neighbors:

There are many children in my family compound, and we read the stories together. Everyone is talking and laughing. It is so joyful. The children say, "This story is for so and so . . . that neighbor who is always beating his children," or "So and so should get this book. I'll read the stories next to her so she can hear them," or "That woman needs to hear this. She is just like the woman in this story." Some neighbors come, watch, and listen to the stories. I invited them though they are not members. My neighbor changed. All her children had sandals, but that child from outside, who lives with her, didn't. All her children had nice clothes, but that child didn't. But now she bought that child sandals. She even combs her hair, but before she didn't.

Rumormongering is a serious source of conflict between spouses as well as between co-wives in polygamous societies. For example, a first wife will sometimes instigate rumors against a second wife because often a husband neglects his first wife after he marries a second. This respondent took action because the story had such personal resonance for her. I heard this comment often—that a story made one feel that the writer had looked into his or her life:

It is as if the person who wrote this has looked into my life with the story of rumormongering. There are two of us . . . me and my co. She makes allegations like saying, "You're acting like this . . . you're not getting our husband to take full responsibility . . . you're trying to get our husband to leave me and my children." None of which is true. I sell things in the market to meet needs for the family. So my co looks at me and thinks that everything is being taken care of by our husband. I called both of them and we sat down and discussed this. She said that our husband is ever buying me clothes and yet the husband is not doing anything for her. I told her, "Look, I sell things in the market and that's how I've manage to get these clothes." I learned there are ways to stop rumormongering unlike before when I used to fight her. She no longer talks against me.

A frequent source of tension occurs when a man takes his wife's produce, sells it at the market, and uses the proceeds for drinking alcohol or other personal uses. Tension is especially high when a husband takes his wife's produce and gives it to her co-wife. Narrative practice helped people reconcile these conflicts:

I'm a hard-working woman, but the man who inherited me is not hard working and the other woman [co-wife] is so careless. They don't store in the granary, and they're always depressed by famine. He carried off my harvest to the other house. Such a thing really hurt me a lot. My co-wife is also in this program and this helped. We no longer hold grudges. We used to hate one another. Nowadays we dig together and he treats our children equally. He kept on telling me when he read the stories, "This thing really touches me. This is like I'm laughing at the death of my own brother. I'm sorry, I won't repeat it." I learned if you reconcile and forgive, you can carry on.

I repeatedly heard *now I know right from wrong*. This phrase was repeated in regards to social as well as to intimate interactions as this person reported:

Those who are not in the program do not accept that forced sex is bad. They say, "When you brought a woman, she is your own and whether you rape her or not . . . whether she wants sex or not, that is not your problem . . . you can do anything you want to her." We have knowledge and skills that people who are not in the program don't have. We know the difference between bad and good.

BECOMING AD HOC COMMUNITY EDUCATORS AND COUNSELORS

Participants took pride in being able to help others. They were called to settle a dispute or to talk to youth or others about what they had learned in the program: "I believe there is a great change in my life—that's why I am respected by the community. If there is a wrangle in the neighborhood and if I intervene, people listen to me. They call me *teacher*. I gained courage to talk about reproductive health, domestic violence, how to educate boys and girls, and how to avoid drinking recklessly."

There were examples of participants talking to someone who they knew was either being abused or was abusing someone else. In this regard, respondents mentioned how those who had been in the program had helped them resolve a conflict:

> So Ajok saw what was going on and asked me if she could mediate. . . . I accepted. My brother-in-law told me that he wanted to inherit me and if I refused he'll pack my things and take them away. Ajok told him it's not good to act that way. You have to negotiate to solve problems. After refusing, my brother-in-law took all my things and distributed them to my relatives and told me, "If you want all those belongings back, you should accept me." I took the issue to the LC (Local Council) and recovered those properties. There's big change because of Ajok. She helped me.

One man asked to speak with the evaluators because he wanted to tell them about his brother. He explained why he was proud of his brother:

> My brother was a drunkard . . . but after he joined this program, he started to reduce his drinking. Before he beat his wife and did other stuff to her . . . he didn't listen to us. I wondered what kind of program made my brother change? So I went to listen. I think this program really teaches good things . . . the group really gives good advice. Now my brother gets up and digs. I was thinking maybe my brother used to be alone and after he joined, he was with his age mates and this made him change. Now his wife is getting fat and she looks happier.

I usually ask, "What prompted you to start this conversation with this particular person?" I want to learn how participants are applying what they learned and under what circumstances. Generally participants talked about seeing a problem and now, because of the program, knowing how to talk about it:

> We have a neighbor who has been clearing his land to prepare it to plant peanuts and we helped him clean his land so he doesn't resort to burning it. We showed him the books and that's what helped me talk to this man and decide to help him. I am very confident now because the program showed me what is right and what is wrong.

BECOMING A ROLE MODEL

Participants talked about becoming a role model. Some felt motivated because of the character of the facilitator: "The facilitator is a role model for me. She is a woman like me and she does not fear. She can talk about anything and this helped to remove the shame and fear within me."

People talked about being role models in their respective communities and being called *mediator* or *teacher*. Some who had not been in the program spoke about seeing a participant as a role model and wanting to be one as well:

I am not a person who usually mistreats children because I know misery is not sweet. I have a girl [*restavek*] who lives with me. When she behaved badly, I used to beat her. Since I started reading the stories, I decided not to beat her anymore. When I see how much misery the children who stay with other families are passing, I, myself, want to be a model.

Some used this new respect (being perceived by the community as a role model) to motivate a husband or wife. They said things like: "You must change your behavior because now that I've been in this program, people expect us [her family and her] to be role models for the community."

Others recognized that program participants had acquired special skills. Women and men who had participated in the program became known as community counselors and were asked to intervene to help others: "They have not been selfish about the knowledge they got. Participants have been encouraging us nonmembers to live by what they tell us. They have been sharing with us how we can end violence."

BUILDING COMMUNITY SOLIDARITY

Two of the environmental program narratives had to do with market conditions. Participants and non-participants reported changes in the market:

Now we do it ourselves. When you are in the market, you see a lot of trash, and before, people would think, "She doesn't clean up. So why should I clean up?" But because they've been in the program, their awareness is high and they clean up and they talk to other people to clean up. They tell people, "You can't wash sugar. So you have to cover your sugar." They got this example from the story about the child who got sick from the dust and microbes in the sugar.

Another market woman stated, "This program is like a booster for us. There is a saying that one person is weak, but together we are strong. In the market now we take our brooms and clean up the whole place."

Actions extended into issues not directly covered in a program. Participants used their skills to settle land disputes, teach children in schools about sexual health, take an active role in community meetings, and help people in their community who were bereft of companionship and support: "They come from different villages and different wards. They weren't in a group before. Because of this program, they really help each other. There is a woman here who has no children . . . she is called Irena. The participants smeared her whole hut (washed the mud floor with a watery mixture that leaves a cement-like surface) and dug in her garden—they never did that before."

People Talk about the Methodologies

Evaluators usually ask participants about their experiences in the learning groups. One frequent comment was about the emotional intensity of the narratives: "At times, we would laugh a lot and jump up and down. At times we cried. The stories gave us feelings of strength and hope."

Participants and facilitators talked about how people laughed during the program meetings. Because the stories are often about people's sexual escapades, participants laughed in part because they had never seen this kind of public exposure of private issues before. "Participants were really happy . . . they wanted to go over the stories again and again . . . they laughed a lot." While the subject matter was serious, through laughter, participants were more able to confront uncomfortable issues:

> However you came from home and have quarreled with someone or your husband . . . when you come here, you will relax and enjoy and forget your problems . . . and when you go back home, you will be so jolly. I have never seen training like this . . . this is the first of its kind to come here because it was so educational and enjoyable.

Participants said the narratives were a reality—"the stories are about our lives." They used words like *amazing, exactly what's happening here every day, they touch your heart.* One person said, "I felt the story from deep inside me . . . from my gut to my toes because it happened to me." Many said that anyone could find something in a program that they could learn from, something they could relate to. Many said that specific stories or characters described their situation: "I have gone through this program, and I have seen the stories talking about the drunkard and they are really about me."

I think narrative credibility is essential to narrative practice. Sometimes I insert this question into an interview, "Who do you think wrote these stories?" I want to find out if people think a native of their country or a foreigner wrote them:

> These books are from a person who sat down and thought "What should the health of a person really be?" That is the person who wrote these books. This is exactly the real story . . . exactly. It happens exactly the way it is in the stories. There is really nothing that is missing. These are the things that we always do within our community. Issues of drinking . . . of sexual intercourse . . . forced sex . . . everything. I don't know who wrote these stories, but I appreciate what this person did because this is something real . . . on the ground. The person must be from here. An outsider wouldn't know these things.

The stories were a means of convincing a reluctant partner that changes need to be made. When a participant took the books to a spouse, many reacted as this man. "Whenever my husband reads, he says, 'They wrote this story as though they know my condition. I think this is so moving.'"

Children also read the stories. Some reacted emotionally to seeing children like themselves being abused, as this child explained: "I saw where they burned the child with a pot. I saw that! I saw where they were mistreating *restavek* children. If I saw that, I wouldn't let that person hit that child! I would grab the stick! I would grab the pot!"

Many people saw the narratives as moral lessons—"It's like reading the Bible." As I said before, "I now know right from wrong" was repeated frequently during the evaluation interviews. While people knew right from wrong before the program, being in a program gave them the confidence and credibility to speak out:

> My husband had a garden and a goat came into his garden and he got mad. He killed the goat. During the program, I showed him the books. I told him, "Killing the animal was not right. That hurt the owner of the goat. You should bring it to a mediator next time." That's what I told him. Now I can say what is right.

This facilitator described how the images together with the text shocked participants, which led to greater awareness:

> They talked about the woman hitting the child with the pot and about children sleeping in the bed while Ester was sleeping on the floor. The way the images reflect life experiences together with the text truly talks about reality. I feel that the text states everything the images are saying. It's important, the combination of both. The stories upset them but now they understand.

I heard repeatedly from respondents that "I know this is the truth because I heard the story" or "I know it's true because I saw the pictures."

Ordinarily I do not write a narrative that compares stark examples of good with bad behavior because I think a narrative with these examples could become overly didactic. However, I wrote a story about two sisters, one sister who treats her servant girl poorly and complains about the girl's bad behavior, and another sister who treats her servant girl well. The story compares the outcomes of the two servant girls' behaviors as a consequence of their different treatments. Participants did not want to be like the bad sister: "I remember the story where one of the aunts was treating her niece well and the other was saying bad things to her niece and hitting her. I buy more stuff for my niece now because I know now that this is my responsibility."

I am interested in finding out how the process of discussing alternative endings for the stories affected participants. A few participants complained about the stories not having endings, but most said, "I believe by the stories not having an end, it gave us so much to think about 'cause you have to think what it would be like. We got suggestions from each other, telling us something you don't know. So we educated each other. We also became better friends."

Participants benefited from being able to share their experiences and hear the experiences of others. I repeatedly heard "I learned I am not the only one." This led to greater self-assurance; as one woman explained, "The program showed us we are unique but our lives are not that different. People kept bringing in new people to hear the stories. Someone shared something very personal and then the next one . . . and the next one opened up. We shared our own stories—gradually, we're gaining the confidence to speak up."

In the combination of a recognizable story with culturally resonant dialogue, participants acquired more awareness and more knowledge, which led to their confidence to speak: "Before this program I had nothing to say. Now I have a lot to say. I feel differently than before. I heard about it, but it was never really broke down for me. The stories are what we were goin' through on a daily basis. I learned it is okay to talk about it . . . what is so horrible . . . what you hide. It's okay 'cause now I know I'm not the only one."

I trained facilitators not to push one point of view or belittle a participant who expressed an idea that others (including the facilitator) did not agree with. Therefore, I am interested in finding out if, during discussions, there were disagreements between participants and how these were resolved:

> Some said if a man comes home drunk and forces you into sex, just accept it . . . because otherwise you will be hurt. But others said, "No, you can't accept it. Why accept it if you don't want it or need it? It's better to manipulate him and give him food and welcome him very well and all that . . . So since he is drunk, he will end up sleeping instead of disturbing you. You distract him." Some said if this happens, a woman should report it to the authorities because this is a violation of our rights.

In some programs there were mixed groups of men and women. This mixed group talked about men beating their wives. The participants disagreed: "People discussed how men beat women and the women said that men can't live on their own. So it is better if a woman is compensated if she is beaten up . . . like in the story when she is given a goat . . . but the men said, 'Maybe the woman is the root cause. So men shouldn't have to give a goat.'"

During any one session, the facilitator asks questions to prompt dialogue between participants. The facilitator also does this to teach participants how and why to ask questions. Participants described this process: "When the monitor asks you questions, you learn to think. Sometimes you don't really understand the question. So then you ask the monitor questions so you understand. We learned how to ask questions."

People spoke about how the role-plays helped them listen to and not distort information. One man said after he acted in a role-play, "This made me feel proud and self-motivated." Many said that acting and watching the role-plays "refreshed our minds so we didn't forget when we went home."

One goal of narrative practice is to encourage retrospection. In this example, the role-play helped a participant reflect on a previous incident in his life and consider how he might change: "I fought with my wife when in-laws said that my wife is in a love affair with another man. They wanted to see how I would react. Later I realized that what I did was wrong and I felt ashamed. Acting the part of Ayena [from the Ugandan story *Rumormongering*] helped me to learn to investigate before taking any action."

This participant described how the role-plays inspired change in a broader way:

> You have the story in the book and the role-play. It is our culture. You are doing things happening in our neighborhoods. When watching or doing the role-play, you can see the positive in your life and the bad. In the role-play we learned how to behave toward others—how we should respect and talk to one another. This kind of role-play really made a lot of changes about how mediation helps to release grievances between two partners. My participation in the role-play taught me to be a good listener.

As one participant said, the important thing is not the stories alone but the stories in engagement with others: "When you are reading on your own, only you are reflecting. When you have several people responding to each other, you act and take the path."

People Talk about Challenges

Ordinarily rural communities are reluctant to have public discussions of explicit sexual issues, particularly when these might involve men and women who are not spouses. The images in the stories vary from suggestive to shocking as this facilitator related:

> When I first saw the books, I thought, "How can I do this training . . . how can I facilitate this? These things are obscene." But I got courage during the training and the same thing happened here. In the beginning people feared but they got courage after going on in the books. They realized these are normal things of humans, and it happens in every house. There's no need to fear now.

In one program in which community health workers thought the materials might draw negative reactions, they organized a group within a political leader's house. By gaining the leader's support, health workers were able to facilitate other learning groups. However the introduction of a program into a community was sometimes problematic:

> The program started out well at the beginning, and then they checked the pictures and people said this program is sorcery and some left the program. I didn't force them. . . . I had to look for other people. I started informing them again about the program. . . . I said this is about violence and sexual health . . . then a few who understood joined the group.

And then sometimes the opposite happened and people unable to participate blamed the organization for not including everyone. One facilitator commented, "Those who had left the group wanted to come back, but I didn't accept them because we had enough . . . the gap had been filled." In some places, a program was conducted in open, public spaces and passers-by would stop, observe, and ask to join when the program was repeated.

In one venue, mothers and daughter-in-laws or sons and mothers were in the same learning group. Putting certain people together in a group where sex was openly discussed was culturally prohibitive. Initially this caused problems, and as a result, some left the group. In one place, participants explained that this conflict almost ended the program, but the facilitator had the wherewithal to divide the group into two. Some husbands, after seeing the pictures, refused to let their wives attend:

> My husband said this program is for widows and prostitutes. I told him this pro-
> gram will help prevent violence, but he said it will increase violence. After joining
> three sessions, my husband threw my properties outside. Then I used the skills
> I'd learned in the program to explain things to him. He gradually understood.
> Now my life is good. People in the program can testify to this. Even my husband
> respects me now.

Sometimes groups of women visited a husband who had refused to let his wife join the program, and they convinced him to allow her to attend.

In some programs there was initial resistance particularly if the program was based in a community rather than in an institution. I learned that the stories with the images should not be seen independently from a program. The response to sexual imagery seen separate from a program was different from the response when seen in the context of a program. In some cases, facilitators, together with local leaders, managed to smooth the way for a program's acceptance. However, I learned that these sensitivities could cast initial aspersions on a program. Once a program began and people learned what a program was really about, negative reactions apparently dissipated, though I do not know if there were other women who were barred from joining or men who refused to join and how many of these there were.

Challenges ranged from getting an alcoholic husband to stop drinking and beating his wife and children to organizing a community to protect fast-depleting resources, as this woman related:

> I saw how to construct *misek* [human-constructed rock or straw barriers to hold
> top soil and water], how to conserve water, top soil, and make fertilizer in the
> books. They talked about burning the fields and worms. I would like to make
> *miseks* but we lack *groupmas* [community groups]. I talk to my friends, but it's
> never done. If the rain doesn't fall now, we can't work on the land. We just wait.

Changing an abusive partner or one that was putting his family at risk was also difficult. This woman had not been able to influence her husband:

> I felt so proud about this program because it talks about domestic violence and decision-making, and I shared this with my husband though he never responded positively. I loved the stories. My husband is too alcoholic and forces me into sex even though the children are still awake, and I try to talk to him, but he never listens to me . . . even when I tell him I'll sleep on the floor without the mattress. When I tried to share the stories with him, he was very rude to me, but I tried my best. My husband goes drinking and returns at dawn. . . . I really feel it is putting my life at risk and each time he comes, he arrives when I am going to the garden and he wants to force me into sex. I feel these books are helping the community a lot . . . a lot.

This woman tried to talk to her husband with the authority of the stories, but she failed to influence him. Changes that she spoke about in the community were not affecting her husband's behavior and the profound risks she was being exposed to. Others as well spoke with pride about how the program was changing the community though they saw little hope in their own situation.

Though less common, a few divorced because of fear of becoming HIV-infected or because of years of infidelities and domestic violence, and a few took on tactics not advocated by the program: "He didn't eat the food I prepared. I said to him, 'I know why because you come from your other woman and your stomach is full because you've been eating good food.' He slapped my face, kicked me, and hit me again. I got a rock and hit him. That was it. He has never hit me again."

Not surprising, there are limitations to what any one program can accomplish as this participant explained about the Northern Uganda program:

> Things went so deeply in people's hearts that they cannot be removed . . . for example, cutting someone with a *panga* . . . kidnapping . . . making people become child soldiers. These things cannot be removed or forgotten . . . they are now in the minds of Acholi people. The kind of killing I've seen . . . I've never seen this in my life. So I can't really remove this out of my mind and this program can't do that either . . . but it really helps us with our future and our children.

Differences in Overall Program Impact

The program environment and the involvement of supporting organizations influenced the impact of narrative practice. The Bangladeshi and Los Angeles programs for Latinos and African Americans influenced individuals and families but had less influence over collective change, whereas the Thai, Haitian, and Ugandan programs achieved both in varying degrees. The narratives in the Bangladeshi program were used in door-to-door HIV prevention with less community dialogue. The nature of marginalized communities in Los Angeles did not allow for widespread collective change. The African American program took place in day and live-in treatment centers and incarcerated participants faced enormous challenges once they left these centers. Some of the learning groups in the Latino program had members who came from distant communities, so the possibility of a collective impact was minimal. On the other hand, when learning groups were conducted in the community center of a large housing project, the Latino program had community effect.

The Haitian and Ugandan programs were implemented in communities, often in open, public spaces. These programs were also connected to supporting organization programs, which had ongoing activities in microfinance, literacy, children's rights, and violence prevention, some with deep roots into these communities. Because of this, participants' attendance was sometimes tied to their involvements in these activities. This was particularly significant if that involvement had to do with economic activities like microfinance, which led to high participant attendance.

If participants did not live together in the same communities, participant attendance often rested on the skills of a facilitator or on the importance of the supporting organizations. In the Latino program, for example, a well-liked elementary school teacher facilitated a learning group with parents of children in the school, and this contributed greatly to participant commitment. Of course in closed communities (treatment facilities), participant attendance was mandatory. Participants in these closed communities were noticeably determined to change their lives once they left these communities. I have no data to indicate whether or not they achieved their intentions.

From what participants reported, once they attended one learning session, they kept coming back because "the stories were so entertaining and engaging." In one treatment center, some participants who had served their sentences and moved on returned each Saturday to hear a story and participate in a learning group until the program ended.

In conclusion, when I consider the accomplishments of community narrative practice, some programs were more collective and more sustainable. These took place where learning groups were conducted within a community and had the backing of a respected organization that was willing and able to support the program beyond its field test.

6 | An Example of Narrative Practice

Toma and Sentana

Narrative community practice is a process that involves ethnographic research, data analysis, the creation of narratives, pedagogy, and evaluation. Though evaluation is not one of the steps of narrative practice, I have included excerpts from the evaluation because it will shed light on the impact of this story and its program. In this explanation of one story, *Toma and Sentana*, from the Haitian HIV and AIDS, sexual and reproductive health program, I have created a visual and textual illustration of the process of narrative practice.

Education is Conversation

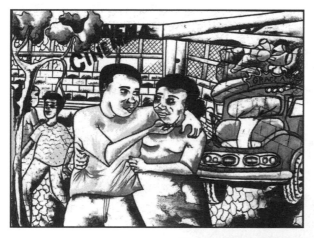

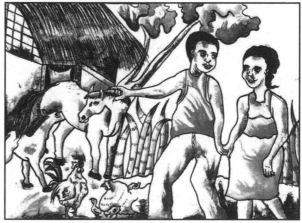

I want to live. We want to live. What about you?

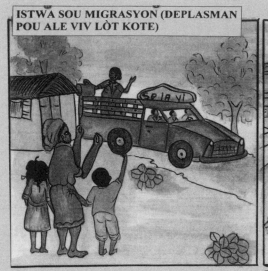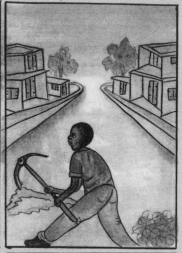

> ISTWA SOU MIGRASYON (DEPLASMAN POU ALE VIV LÒT KOTE)

> Men istwa Toma ak Sentana: Toma wè pa te gen lajan nan kay la pou l ede Sentana oubyen fanmi l. Li deside sòti, konsa li ale Pòtoprens.

> Lè li rive Pòtoprens, li jwenn travay sou wout li. Se te yon travay di. Men tout fason, li te ka fè yon ti lajan pou l voye lakay.

This is the story of Toma and Sentana. Toma sees that he can't earn money to help Sentana and their family. So he decides to leave home to look for work in Port au Prince.

When he gets there he finds a job repairing roads. It is hard work, but it gives him a way to earn money to support his family.

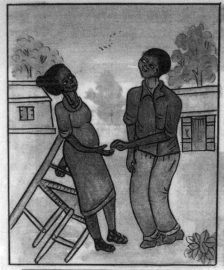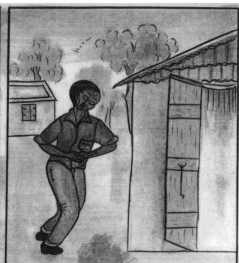

> Nan fen jounen an li te vin fatige epi l te poukont li. Pandan l t apral nan chanm li, li rankontre yon bèl fi ki rele Jaklin.

> Jaklin envite Toma vin nan chanm li an epi yo kòmanse fè lanmou.

When he gets off from work, he's tired and lonely. One day, on the way back to his room, he meets a beautiful woman named Jaklin.

She invites him into her room, and they make love.

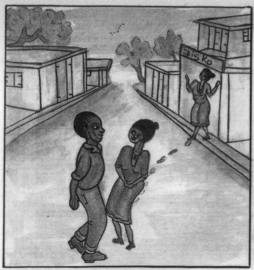

Toma bay Jaklin ti lajan li te fè nan travay li a. Lè lavi a vin bèl pou Toma, li bliye fanmi l.

Kesyon pou brase lide:
Kisa nou panse de istwa sa a?
Kisa nou panse ki pral rive moun sa yo apre ?

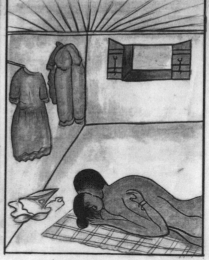

An nou suiv istwa a pou nou wè.

Toma gives Jaklin the money he earns. As his life improves, he begins to forget his family.

What do you think of this story? What do you think will happen now?

Let's keep reading to find out.

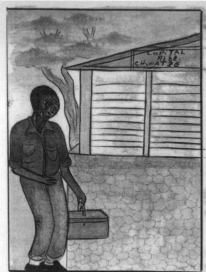

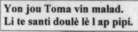

Yon jou Toma vin malad.
Li te santi doulè lè l ap pipi.

Li te deside retounen Dechapèl pou l te ka jwenn tretman pou doulè a.

Pandan Toma nan machin nan, li kòmanse panse ak fanmi l. Li pa t vle pou Sentana konnen li malad. "Woy, Bondye!" Li reflechi epi l di:"Kisa m pral di Sentana ?" Pou kisa Toma te santi l jennen pou l fè Sentana konnen l malad?

One day, Toma gets sick. It hurts when he pees. He decides to return to the countryside to seek treatment. As he heads home, he begins to think of his family. He doesn't want

Sentana to know that he's sick. "What in the world will I tell Sentana?" he says.

Why do you think Toma is afraid to let Sentana know he's sick?

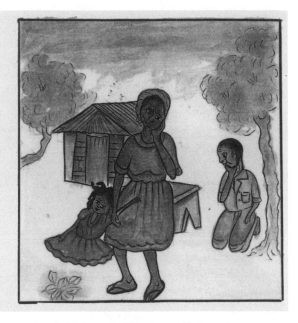

Pandan Toma te Pòtoprens,
Sentana te chita lakay l ap
ret tan lajan paske lajan pou
l fè mache a te twò piti pou
l voye timoun li yo lekòl.

While Toma is in Port au Prince, Sentana sits at home, waiting for whatever money Toma will send. The little money she has *to run her household isn't enough to send the kids to school.*

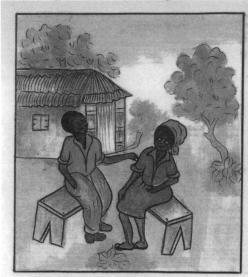

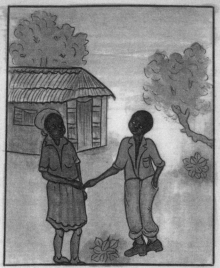

Yon jou Sentana rankontre yon lòt gason
ki rele Pyè. Li te vle ede Sentana nan
pwoblèm li an.

Pyè bay Sentana lajan pou l voye
timoun yo lekòl.

One day, Sentana meets another man, named Pye. He wants to help Sentana.

He gives her money to send her children to school.

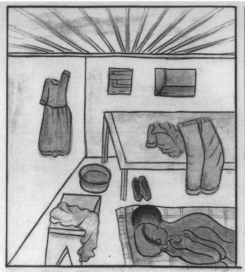

Sa te fè kè Sentana kontan.
Sentana rantre nan chanm li
ak Pyè, epi yo fè bagay.

Sentana is grateful. They go into her room
and make love.

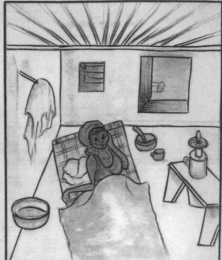

Yon jou Sentana te santi l
malad. Li te mete nan tèt li
petèt Pye ba li yon maladi.
Pandan li te kouche malad
sou kabann li, Toma rantre.

One day, Sentana feels sick. She thinks that
she has caught something from Pye.

While she's lying in bed, Toma walks in.

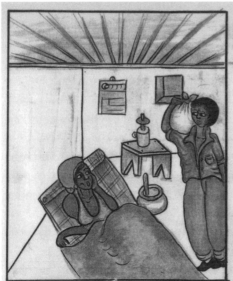

Toma te retounen soti Pòtoprens.
Toma salye Sentana.

Toma has returned from Port au Prince. He
greets Sentana. She's surprised. She wonders
what she can possibly tell him.

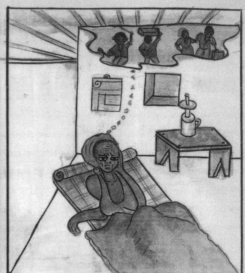

Sentana te sezi lè l wè
Toma. Sentana di nan kè l:
" Woy Bondye!"
" Kisa m pral di Toma?"

"Oh, my God," Sentana thinks. "What if Toma
finds out. What can I tell him?"

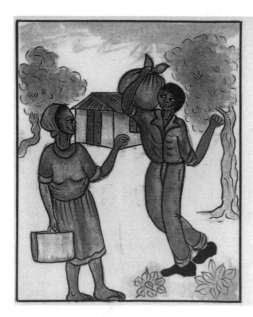

Kesyon pou brase lide:
Eske nou panse Sentana santi l wont?
Pou kisa?
Kisa Sentana ka di Toma?
Kisa Toma ka di Sentana?
Kisa Sentana ak Toma dwe fè ?
Si nou te nan plas Sentana oubyen Toma
kisa nou t ap fè ?
Kisa yon gason ka di mennaj li si l genyen
yon maladi moun pran nan fè bagay ?
Kisa yon fi ka di mennaj li si l genyen yon
maladi moun pran nan fè bagay ?
Ki wòl laperèz ak silans jwe nan istwa
Sentana ak Toma a?
Pou kisa li enpòtan pou youn pale ak lòt sou
pwoblèm yo genyen an?

Questions for Reflection
- *Do you think that Sentana is ashamed of what she's done? Why?*
- *Do you think Toma is ashamed? Why?*
- *What can Sentana say to Toma? What can Toma say to Sentana?*
- *What should Toma and Sentana do? What would you do in their place?*
- *What can men and women tell each other when they have sexually transmitted diseases?*
- *What role do fear and silence play in this story?*
- *Why is it important for us to talk with one another about our problems?*

Ethnographic Research: Introduction

Early on I found an able translator in Rolin, who works for the community education department as a self-styled HIV and AIDS educator. Over the next few weeks we interview over 150 people. In these first interviews I do not use a tape recorder or take notes during the interviews. I fear that people will close up, become focused on what I am doing rather than on what we are discussing. I have a notebook and in between interviews, I jot down reminders. Later these reminders will help me remember conversations from the day. I talk with people across a broad spectrum of ages and years of schooling.

I interview adults and youth alike. The sexual dynamics I see in adults are practiced early on by youth. Some girls complain that some boys are greedy because they refuse sex. These boys tell me they want to focus on their studies. I want to know how men and women begin relationships; why they stay together or separate; what they say to each other when they are angry; what they do when they feel jealous. The word *serious* in the statement "the man was serious" comes up many times in conversations when women describe why they decided to marry. Seriousness equates with the ability and willingness to provide. Many Haitians are in consensual unions. Though they are not officially married, everyone recognizes the couple as such. With this label come obligations. A man may have two or more women living in separate households that he frequents and supports. Many have fathered children with more than one woman, and many women are raising children who were fathered by different men. A man might refer to these mothers as his wives though a casual partner would not have this label. Haitians consider sex a source of health and well-being.

If a man has children with other women, regular distribution is expected. Splitting desire is complicated. Though women expect men's infidelities because, as the Haitian saying goes, "he is a man," men often hide them. Poor families are affected by incremental changes in household resources, and these fluctuations are often sexually related. A man's infidelities might cause anger from his wife but not necessarily abandonment, as long as he continues to provide. However, for a woman, the temporary gain of sex with a man other than her husband might lead to the permanent loss of her husband if he finds out. If a husband has another woman, he might worry that the wife he left behind is clandestinely with another man. I often hear, "Haitians are very jealous people." Given this scenario, how could it be otherwise?

Haitians know AIDS is a disease without a cure. Most know how it is spread, but some say it is a political scheme to stop people from having children. A few feel it is spread by dogs and insects; a few think by consulting spirits, you can find out who has it; a few say by mixing coconut and citrus, you can get rid of it. Some believe in *Zombie AIDS* that is spread when someone takes the bone of a person with AIDS, grinds it into powder, and then infects others. Some say only rich people get AIDS, not poor. I hear this bravado from men, "I have never seen it. If it existed, I would have gotten it."

The following describes the process of ethnographic research, offering examples of interview questions and data and discussing how they are collected. This first step in narrative practice led, in this case, to the creation of *Toma and Sentana*.

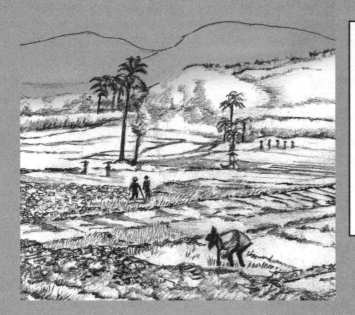

The Artibonite Valley, in central Haiti, is the main rice producing area. The importation of Miami rice decimated local rice production. A few farmers own large tracts of land, but most rent or sharecrop land in the valley or eke out a living in mountains that border this valley. One road runs through this valley, traversing Haiti from Port au Prince in the South to Cape Haitian in the North. In 1995 HIV infection from the valley road to mountain communities ranged from 6 percent to almost none respectively. In the country as a whole, one out of twenty Haitians are HIV positive.

Each day Rolin and I spend hours interviewing people. Sometimes I accompany Rolin to one of his AIDS education talks hoping to corner someone for an interview. After his talk, he asks me how he did. I have deep misgivings. In one church youth sit mesmerized as Rolin simulates male-to-male anal sex gesticulating with a dildo as he talks about the sins of homosexuality. To me it seems surreal. As we walk, Rolin and I talk about homosexuality and abortion. Except for these topics, nothing about sexual health seems to discomfort him. Being trained in the right-wing Protestant church, he is not a proponent of either. I am not trying to reform his religious bents as much as add an alternative health one. We laugh as we talk about our different opinions. Laughter disarms us from backing into corners of judgment without any exit except the dissolution of friendship.

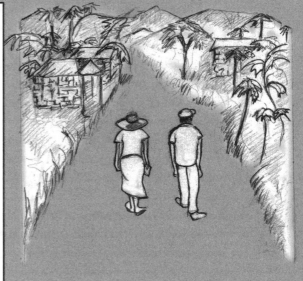

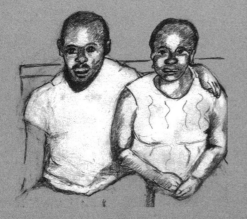

Rolin's wife is jealous. This seems odd to me but not to him. I visit her, bring her things, talk to her in the community education center, and take pictures of her with Rolin. Here is one. I don't want her to worry. Rolin's wife's jealousy intrigues me. Rolin repeatedly tells me, "Haitians are very jealous people." I wonder if this is an expression of love, or a response to the fragility of intimate bonds?

Ethnographic Research: Talking with Women

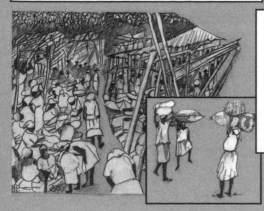

Haitian women control rural markets. Clouds of dust intermingle with hawkers and food stalls. Some women sell sitting on the ground—insistent or reticent, in groups or alone. Some have fresh goods neatly piled, others a few threadbare offerings. Markets are convivial places though not without haggling and an occasional explosion of enraged words. Not a private, quiet place to interview, but a place to observe, to get a sense of things. We meet women on the way, willing to talk if they are not in a hurry to get to the market or home.

I find better, more relaxed conversations visiting women at their homes. Though busy, women will talk while they are working.

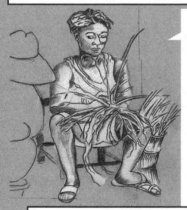

I'm 32, have four children. The oldest is 17. Our parents made us marry. We were very young. I wasn't happy to marry because we were not working, but my father didn't have money. My husband works in the fields and constructs houses. I asked him if he can live with me and he asked me the same. That's what it's all about . . . to look for a better life. If the person loves you, you are obligated to love him too. His blood is with you.

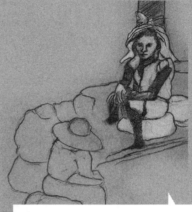

If a man offers money to a woman, she takes it. Women need money so they are always there to have sex. That's how it is. I tell him, "I cannot have sex if I'm hungry."

Do you ever have problems between you?

If I work in the fields and come back home late, my husband asks me, "Where have you been? Why did it take you so long to get back home?" I say to him, "I was working. . . . I had a pig to take care of. So I wasn't pressed to get back. You don't need to be mad for that." Then I make him some coffee I bought with the money I made and he's happy.

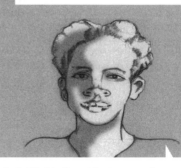

How did you meet your husband?

He sent his cousin to talk to me. My husband works in Port as a mechanic. I didn't believe him because I thought he's a Port kind of guy—a vagabond. I thought he should talk to me, not send someone else. He came. He said he liked me because I'm not into a lot of activities and I go to church. I liked him because I saw he was serious. I asked him for proof that he's a mechanic. He showed me his identity card. Young vagabonds give you words but there's nothing to back them up. Anything I asked him to do, he'd do. I said, "I know you're a guy and you can't stay without having sex." He said he didn't sleep around with a lot of women. I wanted to find out if I didn't have sex, would he leave me. I was really scared about that.

When he comes back from Port, do you ask him questions?

I don't search for the truth. He said, "I have a child now. You're my wife. If you have other women, you have to give them money. The money I have is for you and my child." I don't believe him because he's a guy. They don't give the truth. I just stay with what he tells me. I accept it.

Ethnographic Research: Talking with Women

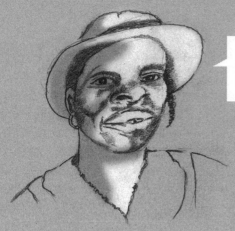

What did you say when you started to live together?

I asked him what he wanted. I said, "If you're with me to play, you can leave because I'm not into games." You know when you get married how things are. He's a man.

What do you mean "He's a man"?

He had other women, but he never lived with them. You can never really trust a guy. I don't get mad. Men are like that—they never stay with one woman. He can be friendly to someone. I won't know what kind of friendship they have. He won't be clear. He'll say the person is not for him, but with experience, I know what's true.

How did you find out he had another woman?

One day he told me something: "She said she would never wash her husband's underwear." I thought, 'What kind of things are they talking about?' He said that was a conversation they were having in the machine [car], but I didn't believe him. After 15 days, he bought a sack of charcoal for her. Then I knew they had a thing together.

Then what did you do?

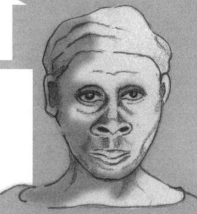

I kept quiet, but one day we were driving, and we saw her on the road. He stopped to talk to her. She tried to talk to me, but I ignored her. When we got home, he asked me why I was so unfriendly. I told him that I wasn't going to talk to his wife. He kept on saying, "It's not true!" I explained, "You make 200 [Haitian dollars] imagine! You have children . . . the whole 200 is not just for you. It needs to be separated and there's never going to be enough!" He was obligated to end it.

He was working in construction in Port au Prince. He didn't come back. While he was gone, I didn't have other men. I think he had other women. I had little money in my hands.

What did you do?

I didn't want an argument. He didn't want to take care of the children. I gathered all his things and put them outside. I called him before the courts. He gave me money. After that, he returned. Now we don't have any problems. Where there's meat, is there anger?

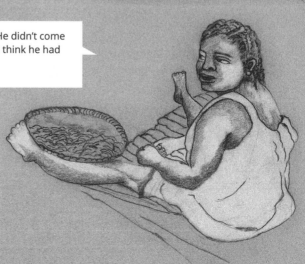

Ethnographic Research: Talking with Women

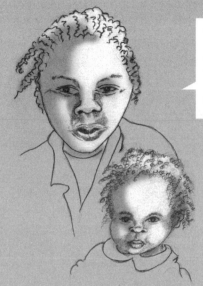

There's money and it should be only for you, but he's sharing that money with other women. He says the money he gives to other women is nothing . . . I shouldn't be bothered. Women are bad. They just attach themselves to him. He always says she's a cousin. He has money. So if he's not having sex with other women, they'll say that he's not a man.

What do you say?

You just can't say anything. Men cannot stay with just one woman. If women did it, they would speak badly of you. . . . I'm jealous for money. I stay with him for the children. He has a child with another woman. It's a problem for me if my children need something and I can't find him. I was the one who was here before her anyway.

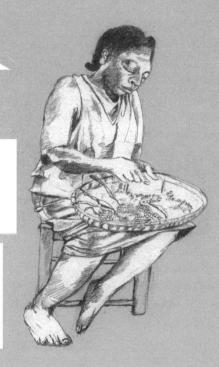

He had many women and children and he gave them what I worked to get. He didn't want me. He said, "You don't have the right to say anything to me." He wouldn't listen to me. So I just stayed by myself and worked to raise my two children. I did it all by myself. And then, after all that time . . . after 11 years . . . he brought all his clothes and hung them on the wall. He came back.

What did you do?

What could I do? It's his house. I couldn't put him out. I just ignored him. He told me, "You are my wife." When I made food, I gave him a little . . . coffee, bread, banana. I washed his clothes. I took care of him because if I didn't, people would think badly of me. I was obligated, but I had closed my heart off to him.

What did you say to him?

I told him, "See, you never imagined you would turn into an old man with no money and women would not want you anymore!" He said, "Oh, let's not talk about that." He doesn't have other women. Women ask for money, and if you don't have any, they won't care about you. We don't argue. We don't really talk. We just live our lives and do what we need to do.

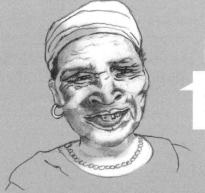

Her husband left her to go to Miami many years ago.

I remember him all the time and I know he remembers me. There's nothing I'd hide from him. If he has such a disease, I would get it because I'd let him do whatever he wants.

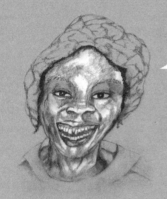

You see women fighting over men. When my husband goes out, I don't know where he goes and I can't say anything. But when I return from the market late because I couldn't sell anything, he says, "You were with another man." We fight. Jealousy makes you feel small . . . you don't want to eat . . . you don't feel okay.

I interview an HIV and AIDS counselor at the hospital.

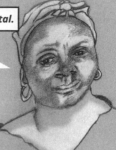

Men say, "I am a man therefore I can find other woman," . . . but if they know a woman has another man, they will break her neck. Once I told a man during counseling to bring his wife. He told me, "I am not alone. There are three more." Then all four came together.

What happens when one of you wants sex and the other doesn't?

If I tell my husband, I don't want to have sex, he still does it. When he insists, I do it. If I don't want to, he says it's because I have another man. I must satisfy his needs. I think if a woman refuses sex, the man will leave her. People have relationships for money. If a woman is with another man, her husband can beat her very hard—next to death.

If your husband sees you talking to another man, what does he say to you?

He says, "That person was talking to you a lot. It wasn't about charcoal you were talking." I don't listen. I am scared because he's suspicious. First there's a lot of talk and then he beats me. Then we cannot talk at all.

I hear the unexpected.

If a woman isn't good . . . if she has many partners, the husband should correct her. It's the same for your children when they don't act well. If you talk to them and they don't listen to you, you hit them. Some women like being hit. A man shouldn't normally whip a woman, but if she does something bad and she doesn't listen to him, he should whip her.

How does your husband show he is angry?

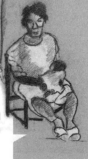

The first one was bad. He hit me. He didn't love me. He wouldn't let me go out. He said that if a car hit me, he would have to come and take my body. He said he is a guy and it's him that's supposed to tell me what to do. If he saw me talking to a man, he would hit me. Everyone told him he didn't have the right to do that. I didn't have other men.

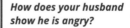

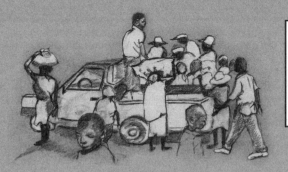

I see men at the market loading and unloading tuk-tuks (pick up trucks that transport people and goods). Men care for large animals, plow fields, carry heavy loads of charcoal (as do women) and wood, construct things, and repair roads. I also see men loitering, playing the lottery, talking, and waiting in anticipation of something.

There are many hard working farmers.

I don't have sex with my wife anymore though I tell her to behave herself. Women are very careful because they get pregnant and men do not. It's that simple. But my wife isn't hot. She would be scared to have sex with me if she thought I had a sexually transmitted disease. If she gave me a sexually transmitted disease, I'd leave. I'd think she no longer cares about me.

Sometimes men are difficult to interview— more interested in exhorting platitudes than in divulging personal information.

Even if a husband takes care of his wife with money, he has to come back and give her sex. If you're out for a long time, you feel she needs sex. It's the same for the man. If he doesn't find love from his wife, he'll go to another woman. If their communication is bad, everyone will do whatever they want.

You can't catch a woman. It's easier to catch a rat. You never know where women go. Certain women accept intercourse with different men and get diseases. Women are the worst. When men from the Dominican Republic came here, many women got pregnant. Some women go North and South selling goods. Market women have sex when they travel.

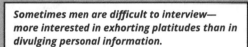

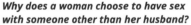

Why does a woman choose to have sex with someone other than her husband?

Times are hard. Prices are very high. Women used to find ways to make money. For 10 *gourde* [25 cents US] women aren't going to buy a condom. Women are looking for money. So there are obligations to accept sex. When you have lots of money like a driver, hougan [Voodoo priest], or a doctor, you can have lots of women. Girls look for older men with money. They need school fees and nice clothes. A girl might go to an adult for counsel. It's not good because she doesn't use condoms, but it's good because he gives her money. If a man's got a big butt, he calls a girl, "Come live with me."

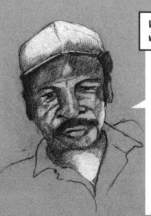

Ethnographic Research: Talking with Men

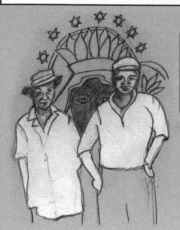

I visit Voodoo priests at their temples. They probably know the most about sexual behavior since they are usually the first people consulted for sexual and reproductive problems. During one visit, I talk to a priest and his client, an old man who lives by himself. He tells me his children are trying to stop him from taking a woman into his house.

My children try to stop me from having sex. I have sex with women in the mountains. I don't use condoms with these women there because they don't have AIDS. In Port people have AIDS but not in the mountains. It will never come there.

How do you know that?

Because city people have no attraction to people who live in the mountains.

The medical doctors tell me that priests have sex with their clients. What do you think about that?

You know who has sex with their clients—doctors from the hospital! Why else are they driving up and down visiting clients? Of course . . . priests . . . doctors . . . only a few do this. Maybe more of the *bokors* [evil doers] do this—not the *hougans* [natural healers].

What kinds of sexual problems do people come to you for?

Many women come because their husbands are unfaithful. This is private. I help her with magic. I call the spirit and it ties up the husband's spirit. The husband may have many women but after he is tied up, he cannot go out. I give his wife a charm to give him so that he will not see other women. Then he is only interested in his wife.

What about when a man suspects his wife?

I give the man magic powder to put in his wife's navel. When she has intercourse with another man, the man does not know, but he receives the powder. Afterwards, he becomes sick. I call the spirit and the spirit makes the diagnosis. I don't do anything myself. I put herbs, rhubard, cocksui, and green kalbas in water. A client drinks it. This *refreshi* is for syphilis and gonorrhea. It can be used for reproductive tract infections, pain at intercourse, and burning urination. Symptoms for men and women are the same.

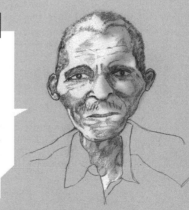

Ethnographic Research: Talking with and about Youth

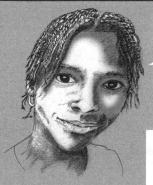

Why do you love your boyfriend?

He has a lot of respect for me and he helps me. When someone likes you, he studies your body and then calls you to ask you a question. When you don't like the way a boy talks to you, you leave him. If he has other girls and you don't want him, you say, "Let's do it tomorrow." One day this boy told me he loves me. We had sex at his house secretly.

When you have a girlfriend, it's serious. You try to know what she's doing, but with a friend, you don't care. A friend is just for sex. I have only one girlfriend but I meet other girls. They live close by. Sometimes they are the ones I go to school with—I have many.

I ask adults how they feel about the sexual behavior of youth.

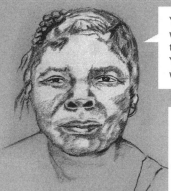

Young people don't listen to their parents. This is different than when we were young . . . we didn't have sex until 25. Sometimes parents arranged the relationship. Parents were strict. Today you see the way they walk. Young girls are not careful. They stand on the street . . . talk to anybody . . . wear very short skirts and t-shirts. It's like they're naked.

There are no activities to keep youth busy. I have a little sister. She can leave in the morning and not come back until late at night. I was never like this. Parents now have too many troubles. Kids want nice clothes, but the parents can't buy them these things. They are too poor. Life was not so hard before. Parents should educate their kids.

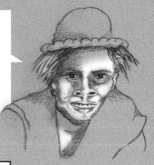

Why do relationships between boys and girls end?

My girlfriend wanted things I couldn't afford. It's not good if my girlfriend has several boyfriends or if she asks me for something and I cannot give it to her. Sometimes girls try to seduce me by offering me gifts. Girls don't want a boy who has no work. If you don't give money, girls don't love you. My parents are poor. They want me to study in school. My parents told me that other boys were sleeping with my girlfriend. I loved her very much. In the beginning, I didn't believe it. At the end, it was sad. It was true.

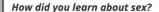

How did you learn about sex?

I had my first sex when we were playing in the water. It just happened. I learned about sex by doing it. You hear about it everywhere but you don't learn about it from parents. My parents tell me "Don't have sex at your age." They just warn me. Most of us have boyfriends and girlfriends, but our parents don't know about this.

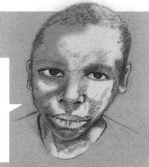

Data Analysis and Writing a Composite Narrative

Toma and Sentana is a simple and straightforward story in plot and dialogue. Narrative desire is first expressed in Toma's desire to find work to feed his family. Thus he travels from his rural home to a city. Once Toma has money, he desires sex with Jaklin, and he forgets his obligation to send money to Sentana. This is a commonplace story, a public narrative. Women respondents consistently talked about their fear of loss of income and sex because of this scenario.

However, what is less publicly told is this story: while household resources decline because a husband is giving money to and having sex with a woman other than his wife, his wife might be doing the same with another man. This is the under-story. In interviews with men, they said they feared this possibility. Factor the odds—if many men are having sex with women other than their wives, whom are they having sex with but other married women whose husbands are doing the same thing?

This narrative is structured so that the public story of Toma's relationship with Jaklin is juxtaposed against the under-story of Sentana's relationship with Pye. While Toma's infidelity is expected, what is less expected is Sentana's. Sentana is the good rural wife waiting for Toma to send money. When Toma does not send money, Sentana meets Pye and he pays school fees so that Sentana can send her children to school. Sentana has sex with Pye and she acquires an STI. Toma suddenly arrives. He also has an STI.

This is a shame-filled narrative. Toma feels shame—he has not met his obligations and is sick with an STI. Sentana might humiliate him. Sentana feels shame because she defied what it means to be a good woman and now risks abandonment if Toma finds out. She could be humiliated.

The narrative is contextualized so that a person who is not literate can easily tell the story. Toma and Sentana's shameful feelings are illustrated in the fears of what might happen if they are found out. At the end of the story, there is no resolution to Toma and Sentana's problems. Instead the participants will discuss and act out these problems. The narrative closes with the question, "What can Toma and Sentana say to each other?

The following describes the practice among Haitian women attending one learning session that focuses on the story *Toma and Sentana.*

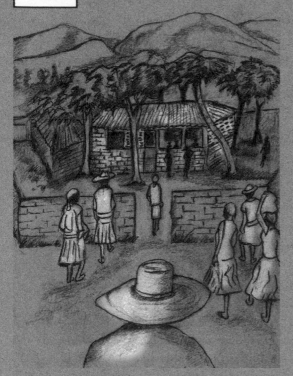

The day is sizzling hot. Without wind, there is a sweltering stillness. Every movement is a slow dance. A tree or building—the only places that offer temporary respite from the sun's intensity. Some women have quietly arrived; others are still walking to the learning center. A fine powder, the dust of a scorched earth, outlines their feet and their leathered soles. Some have come from a market. Relieved, they put down their heavy loads. Others have come from remote places, an hour or more walk. This is rural Haiti. Walking long distances is a way of life. Around the center, the grass is overgrown. One goat grazes while others rest, too hot to chew.

The women greet each other.

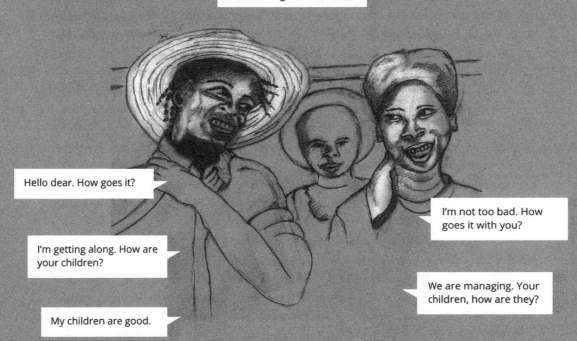

Hello dear. How goes it?

I'm not too bad. How goes it with you?

I'm getting along. How are your children?

We are managing. Your children, how are they?

My children are good.

Friends casually talk with each other. Most are wearing a headscarf or a hat and a newly pressed modest dress. The monitor encourages them into the learning circle. Benches with rough edges, chairs with broken backs, stools with missing legs are randomly placed facing the monitor. What is available is adjusted and steadied as the occupant takes her place. Lateness is not an issue. There are enough present to begin . . . more will soon arrive. The monitor welcomes everyone.

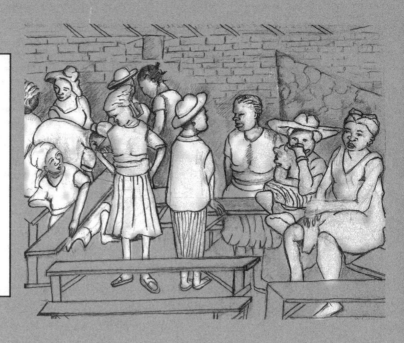

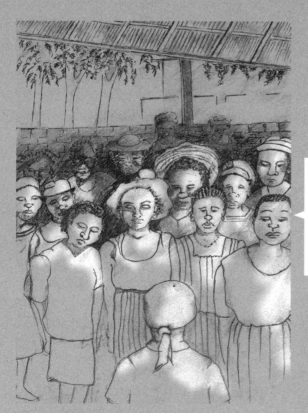

Then everyone stands to say a prayer. Most meetings in Haiti begin with a prayer. Consensus is achieved in: "We are all here under the benevolence of a higher power."

Let us pray to God who watches over us.
God almighty, give us light. Protect us from evil.
Thank all the people who created this program for us.
God, we are your servants. You are our master.
In our blessed savior's name, Jesus,
God's son, and in God's name.
Amen.

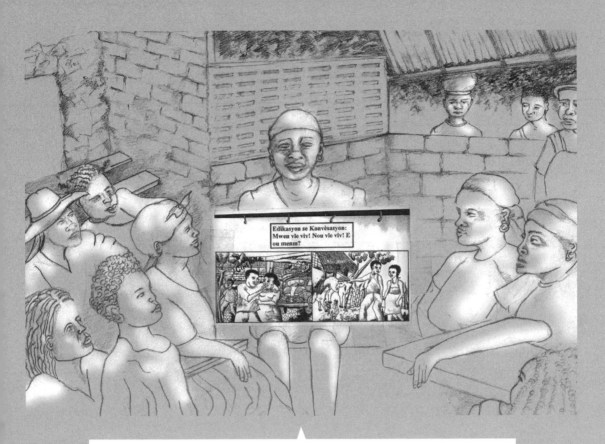

Welcome! I hope you are all well. I am happy to see you. Today we will read the first story of the program, *Education is a Conversation: I Want to Live! We Want to Live! Don't You?* In each session I will read a story and we will discuss it and act it out. This program is very important because here you will learn about sex, sexuality, and sexual diseases and how to prevent them. In this program, education is a conversation, a conversation that you can take to others who are not in this program. From what you learn here you can help your family and friends improve their health. Fonkoze hopes the ideas you learn here will not stay here but spread to others. If you learn private things about someone in our group, please, this information is confidential and should not leave this group. If you attend all the sessions, you will get a certificate showing you completed the program and that you are an advocate for sexual and reproductive health. I hope you continue and receive a certificate. Let's begin the first story.

The monitor asks the following questions: What do you see in this picture? How do you think the people in this picture feel? How do you feel when you look at this picture? Do you see any problems in this picture? And the participants answer.

I see a man on a *tuk-tuk*.

He looks worried.

I feel sad when I look at him.

He is thinking about a woman. Maybe this woman and he had a fight. She is jealous.

Maybe he is running away from a woman.

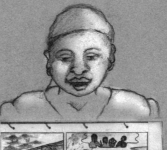

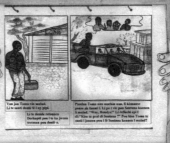

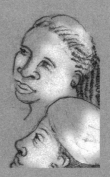

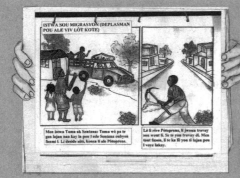

The monitor begins to read the story.

Here is the story of Toma and Sentana. Toma sees there isn't any money in the house to help his wife Sentana or his children. So Toma decides to leave home to look for work in Port au Prince. When he arrives in Port au Prince, Toma finds work repairing roads. It is hard work. But anyway, he has a little money to send home to his family.

The monitor continues to read.

At the end of the day, Toma is tired and lonely. Then one day, on the way back to his room, he meets a beautiful woman named Jaklin. Toma feels happy to meet Jaklin.

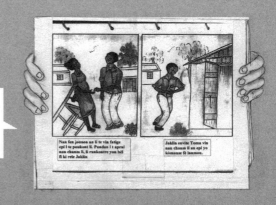

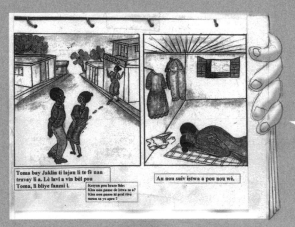

Toma bay Jaklin ti lajan li te fè nan travay li a. Lè lavi a vin bèl pou Toma, li bliye fanmi l.

An nou suiv istwa a pou nou wè.

Kouyon pou louvre lòde: Kisa nou panse de istwa sa a? Kisa nou panse ki pral rive moun nan yo agen?

The monitor asks questions. These questions are not answered but provoke reflection and retrospection.

Jaklin invites Toma into her room and they make love. Toma gives Jaklin money from his job. When life gets good for him, Toma forgets about his family. What do you think of this story? What do you think will happen now? Let's read and find out.

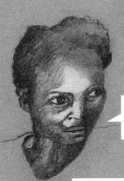

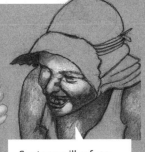

When you are living with a man at home, you never know he won't do the same thing as Toma . . . he . . . men will never tell you the truth.

This is what Jaklin is there for. Toma is a man. This is what men do. My husband would do the same thing.

One day Toma feels sick. He has pain when he pees. He decides to return to the countryside to get treatment. As he heads home, Toma starts to think about his family. He doesn't want Sentana to know that he is sick. Toma worries, "Oh God, what will I tell her?"' Why do you think that Toma is afraid to let Sentana know that he is sick?

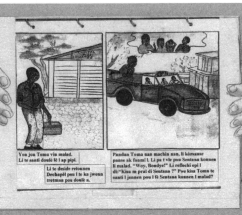

Yon jou Toma vin malad. Li te santi doule lè l ap pipi.

Li te deside retounen Dechapèl pou l te ka jwenn tretman pou doule a.

Pandan Toma nan machin nan, li kòmanse panse ak fanmi l. Li pa t vle pou Sentana konnen li malad. "Woy, Bondye!" Li reflechi epi l di:"Kisa m pral di Sentana ?" Pou kisa Toma te santi l jennen pou l fè Sentana konnen l malad?

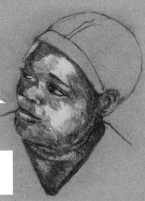

Sentana will refuse sex with him. She will shame him.

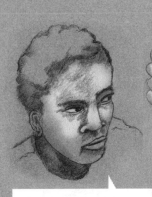

This Toma is a vagabond. He forgets his family. When my husband has money in his pocket he takes other women. He lives in his own head.

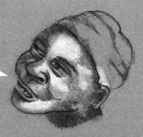

I won't ask him to leave . . . this is the reality. My husband tells me he has the right to do what he wants. He doesn't have another place to eat— only here. I would give it to him.

While Toma is in Port au Prince, Sentana sits at home, waiting for whatever money Toma will send. The little money she has to run her household isn't enough to send the kids to school.

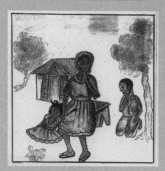

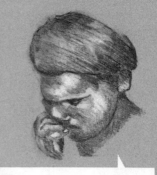

This story is about my life. . . .

One day Sentana meets a man named Pye. Pye wants to help Sentana with her problems. Pye gives Sentana money to send her children to school.

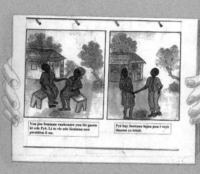

Sentana needs money . . . Toma has left her in misery. She was obligated to find another man. This happened to my sister.

Sometimes you just see money first. Sentana needed money . . . if a man helps you, this is expected.

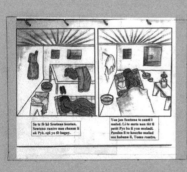

Sentana is grateful. She goes to her room with Pye. They make love. One day Sentana feels sick. She thinks maybe Pye gave her a sickness. While she I sick in bed, she hears someone . . . in walks Toma!

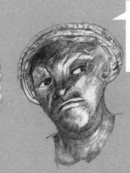

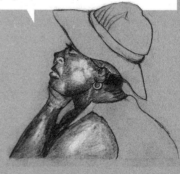

This story is painful for me. This happened to me. My husband says he can do what he wants. You feel you are not a person in the house.

Toma greets Sentana. "How goes it?" Sentana greets Toma, "I am not so bad. How about you?"

"Oh my God," Sentana thinks. "What if Toma finds out. What can I tell him?"

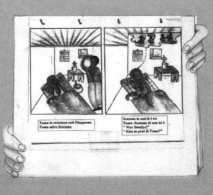

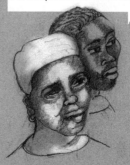

Practice: Collective Retrospection and Interpretation

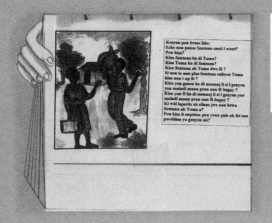

Now the monitor asks discussion questions:
What should Sentana and Toma do?
What can they say to each other?
What can a man tell his wife if he has a sexual disease?
What can a woman tell her husband if she thinks she has a sexual disease?

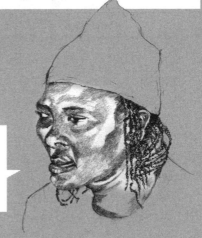

If he tells her, Sentana will say very bad words to Toma. She will refuse sex with him. For me, when Toma came home, I would not accept him . . . because he traveled to work and never sent me money. I would never welcome him home.

They must go to the hospital but they cannot go together. Sentana must go secretly to the hospital. If she tells Toma, he will beat her.

She can try to caress him . . . make him feel good . . . to convince him to use a condom. She needs money from him.

He won't want sex because he is sick. Sentana will wonder why he doesn't want sex with her.

I can't talk about these things with my husband.

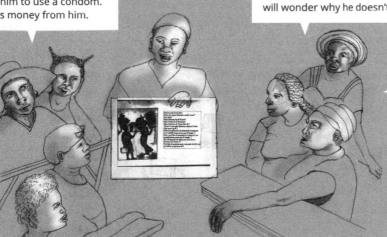

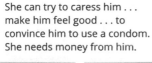

People will see her at the hospital. They will gossip . . . spread rumors. Toma will find out. Someone will tell Toma about Pye.

I won't ask him to leave—it's better to have a man around to raise children. If he has money and you need it . . . even if that man is sick, you shouldn't care about that. I would risk my life and not think of dying.

161

Practice: Sharing and dialogue

The monitor asks, "If you were in Toma and Sentana's place, how would you feel? What would you do?"

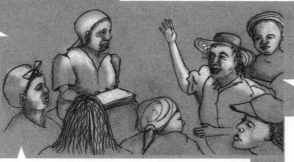

I have a husband who doesn't protect himself. Someday I will get AIDS. He never listens to me. He does what he wants.

My life is like Sentana. My husband left me seven years ago. I never heard from him. He never sent anything to help me and the children.

I would try to talk to him. I don't know what I would say but I would try.

Once I followed my husband and went to the house where he was with this woman. I made a lot of noise outside. The neighbors came. I threatened to burn the house down. He stopped going to that woman's house.

My husband never brought money to feed the children. That's how I knew about him. Then I didn't see him anymore.

The monitor asks, "What do Toma and Sentana fear? Why are they silent? Why are we afraid and silent in our own lives?"

If we keep silent, then we are all in danger. I would try to talk to him sweetly . . . try to encourage him . . . caress him.

I fear my husband would leave me. He would call me a whore. He would beat me. Because of his jealousy, once I had to threaten my husband with a rock to stop him from beating me.

My husband is very jealous . . . when I return from the market late. He says, "You were with another man." For this, he would kill me.

What about asking him to use a condom? Sit down and tell him jokes . . . stories . . . say, "I'm not refusing you because I don't love you."

But if Sentana says she doesn't want to do it, Toma will say she has another man. Then they will fight. He might beat her.

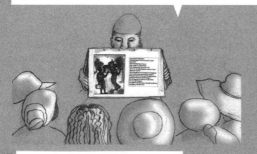

Men don't like to use condoms.

How can she refuse? They are both supposed to want it.

Neither do women.

I keep my body hard so he knows I am not interested in sex.

Practice: The Role-Play—Practicing Negotiation

We are going to have a role-play about Toma and Sentana.

Let's act out the time when Toma walks in on Sentana after he has been away in Port au Prince. As Toma, think about how you will explain yourself to Sentana. As Sentana, think about how you will talk to Toma. Who will volunteer to start the role-play?

I will be Toma.

I will be Sentana.

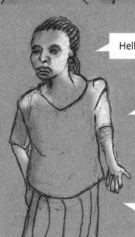

Two volunteers begin the role-play

Hello Sentana. How are you?

Not so bad and you?

I'm managing.

What brings you back without warning?

I was thinking of you. I was lonely for the children.

Do you know we live in misery! You left me six months ago. You sent nothing! Do you think I am a dog in the road?

Please Sentana . . . I, too, suffered . . . life is so expensive in Port. I had to keep alive to come back. Did I not send you money?

The money was not enough. Oh . . . so you have suffered? You look well. You have suffered with your whores! Is that how you suffered?

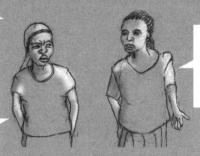

Oh, Sentana . . . how can you say these things?

We barely had food. I didn't have school fees. How was I to send the children to school? What if we had become sick . . . then what? We are in misery here.

Now we must forget all that . . . am I not a man? I had needs. You are my wife, Sentana. I came back to you.

And me . . . am I not a woman?

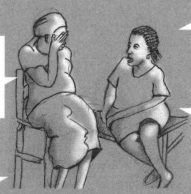

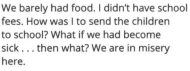

163

The monitor asks the actors to stop at this point and begin again. She suggests that Toma and Sentana try a different line of reasoning.

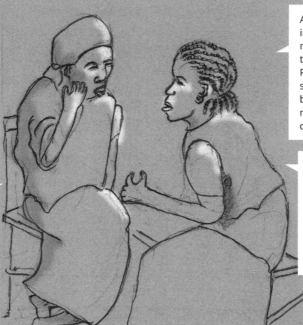

After I arrived in Port in the beginning, I had money to send you. But the longer I stayed in Port, the less able I was to send you money. I have been longing for you, my wife. Where are the children?

The children are in school. Did you have other women? Tell me. There is AIDS out there. Have you thought about that? Do you want to kill us . . . your wife and children? Don't you know you can bring me a disease?

How can you ask me these questions? Do you think I am a child . . . that I don't know how to protect myself? How do you know these things? How do you have money to pay school fees?

At this point, someone from the audience taps the current actor, who is playing Sentana, on the shoulder. That actor leaves her role as Sentana and joins the audience. A new participant takes the part of Sentana.

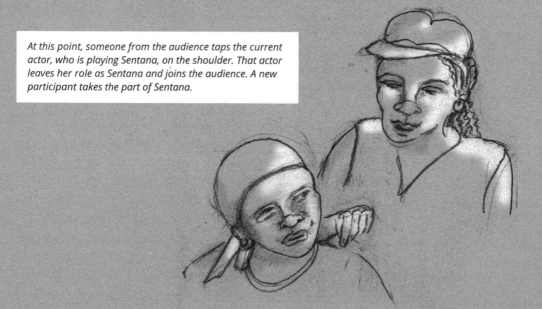

Practice: The Role-Play—Practicing Negotiation

As the role-play progresses, the actors try to find compromise.

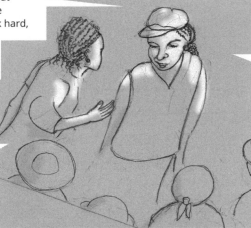

I went to the market. I sold what we had. Do you remember the conditions? I work here. I work hard, but look how we live. I borrowed money from a lender.

Why should I not know about these things? People talk about AIDS all the time. Do you think we are nothing? We were hungry. You are my husband, but we lost you. I was worried about what had happened to you. Do you think I don't care about you?

Sentana . . . please . . . you are my wife. I've come a long distance. I need rest. I'm not feeling well. Please let me rest.

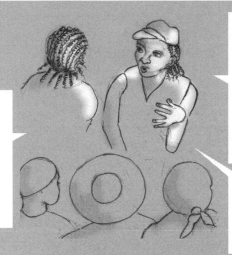

You can rest . . . but first hear me. There was a man here who died of AIDS who infected his wife. Like you, he worked in Port au Prince. Do you think I don't think about these things? If we become sick with AIDS, we will be humiliated. You are my husband and I do not want you to get sick. But when I don't hear from you for so long, what am I to do?

I am here with you. Let us not think about the past . . . we must live again as husband and wife. We were not together before. Now we are. You are my wife. I don't want you to become sick.

Should you not use a condom? I do not know where you have been . . . who you have been with. You know I know you can't stay without going to other women.

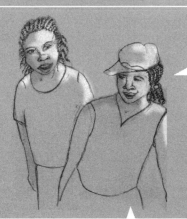

You know I don't have any problem with you, but it is not sweet when a man uses a condom.

I'm not refusing you because I don't love you. But I think we can go to the hospital.

Why? Are you sick? I will go to the hospital . . . since it is me that is feeling sick. Not you.

To get a test for AIDS.

Why do we need a test, Sentana?

We must not be afraid of each other . . . this will make things worse for us. God knows what you have done. Now you must care for your family and give us what is ours. Why should I not take this test? Am I not a woman with needs as well?

165

The monitor asks: What did you learn from this role-play?

I think when Sentana talked sweetly to Toma, she encouraged him. Sugar works better than hot pepper sauce with men. I think when she told Toma she cared about him, Toma was more at ease. Then he could listen.

Men don't like to be accused. When Toma said she was treating him like a child . . . that's what my husband would say. He might get angry and leave the house then.

Without communication, everyone in a family goes their own way.

If a man won't listen, then what do you do? What if he refuses to use condoms with women outside? He might say AIDS does not exist. My husband goes out and I know he goes to meet other women because he dresses up. I tell him, "I need to talk to you because you are the only friend I have." He doesn't listen.

Sentana needed to keep talking to him . . . questioning him . . . in a sweet way. She could caress him. When I do this with my husband, he is more likely to listen to me.

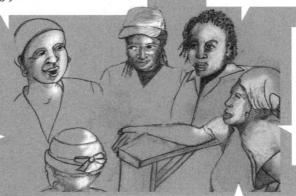

I think Sentana said things that will make Toma suspicious. I know my husband would beat me if he thought I had sex with another man.

The monitor asks: What did you learn from this role-play?

I think it was good to suggest Toma use a condom. Toma might agree because he was sick. But when I was acting as Toma, I couldn't agree with this because this isn't what a man would say. Toma would be suspicious if Sentana asked him to use a condom.

I liked it when Sentana suggested going to the hospital. If they both got a test together, it would be good. I think if I was Toma, I could agree to this.

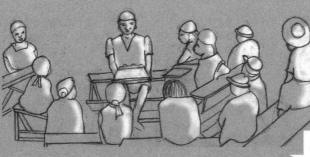

I think in the future I would give him condoms when he leaves home. Then he will know I know what he is doing and he will know that I want to protect the family. Men care about their children. I'm showing him I care about him.

I felt I should not react to Toma. When you react angrily, it only makes things worse. I should ask questions in a friendly way. That's what I tried to do.

We must ask questions. If women don't know how to talk about these things, nothing will change.

If I could show my husband *Toma and Sentana* . . . that would convince him . . . my husband needs to see this program.

I think we should give men condoms; when they travel, they should have condoms in their pocket.

I have not talked about these things before. I'll will try.

It's not easy for a woman to talk about these things.

A friend visited me. He used to be in love with me and wanted to marry me. I told him "I'll have sex with you if you use a condom." He didn't want to. So we didn't have it.

We must talk to them in a way that won't make them angry or suspicious of us. A man must be motivated.

The monitor concludes and everyone stands to pray before they leave.

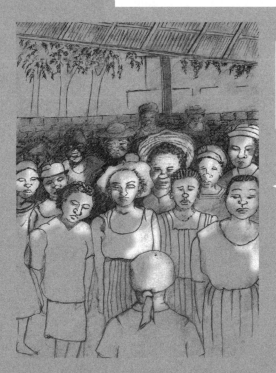

We are learning how to change how we live. We can talk with people to improve our and their lives. We are learning to talk about some issues that cause us shame. By talking and by sharing this education, we will help ourselves and others.

We thank our Lord for this education program Fonkoze has given us. We have more information to share with our families and friends. We have more knowledge to improve our lives. We thank God for bringing us this program to help us. Amen.

Evaluation

For the qualitative evaluation, evaluators interviewed fifty participants (thirty-eight women and twelve men) out of one hundred program participants, as well as all the facilitators and a sampling of children, friends, and neighbors of participants. Because many of the evaluators were involved in the initial research and facilitator training, they noticed participants' behavior had changed. They told me that participants were more self-assured: "They've talked to people outside the program about things they had never talked about before; people in the community contacted people who had been in the program for advice." For both women and men participants the phrase "I am more confident" came up repeatedly.

Men talked about how they appreciated the program. One woman commented that her husband never missed a meeting. "He always wanted to be on time . . . this means it's something my husband really likes." I think one reason the men liked the program was because it gave them the chance to talk about sex in a respectable health program. I know the issue of sexual refusal and forced sex came up during their meetings because without any prompting, men brought these issues up during the evaluation interviews. One man said, "I'm really happy you included men in this program."

I think women's-only or men's-only sexual and reproductive health and HIV prevention programs are blindly pursuing an alien view of heterosexual relations as though men and women pursue sex independently of one another. This strange view negates that these are cultures of *we*. Lack of recognition of the nature of men and women's reciprocity might be causing undue harm. The question an HIV and AIDS program or any program that involves sexual health problems, violence, or other emotionally changed issues should be, "How can people live healthier or better lives, both collectively and individually, within the harnesses of their culture?"

The following excerpts from the evaluation interviews highlight the impact of *Toma and Sentana* and the Fonkoze HIV and AIDS program.

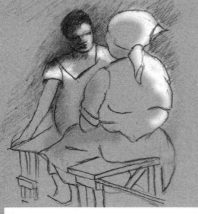

I feel I have something else in me . . . something changed in my heart. I talk to my husband much more. I have more confidence. There are some words I couldn't use before. Now I tell him things like, "When you leave and have other women, take condoms please. I don't want you coming back and bringing me what you got from other women." My daughter now feels she can talk to me. My husband says, "You've changed. You must be learning something in that program."

I really love this program because I learned things I didn't know before. I talk to my children differently today than I did in the past. I tell them how to talk to people. I learned how to ask my husband questions. After hearing *Toma and Sentana* I told my daughter, "Because your husband goes to Port, you can ask him how many people he had sex with. You can say, 'I don't know how many women you've had sex with, but you need to use a condom.'"

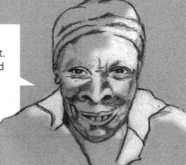

My husband said, "This is a really good program! It's good because as a man, I could tell you that you are the only one I have and then I would have someone else." I asked him, "Why would you have someone else?" He said, "You know I'm living far from you." I said, "I understand—so because you have this mind, if you ever have to do it, use a condom." And, he said, "Not all women like it when a man puts a condom on." And, I said, "If a woman does not want you to put on a condom, don't have sex with her—you don't know what disease she has." Now he is more afraid of AIDS than he was before.

My husband asked, "Where did they find the things in this book?" He changed. Sometimes now, if he has a woman outside, he tells me he used a condom. Before, he would not use one. Now if he uses condoms he has, he comes back with new ones. The program helped me understand a lot of things. He answers me and listens to what I say. I feel very comfortable now. I feel strong.

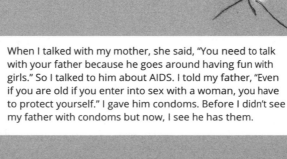

When I talked with my mother, she said, "You need to talk with your father because he goes around having fun with girls." So I talked to him about AIDS. I told my father, "Even if you are old if you enter into sex with a woman, you have to protect yourself." I gave him condoms. Before I didn't see my father with condoms but now, I see he has them.

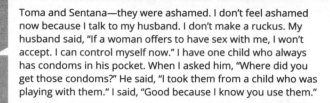

Toma and Sentana—they were ashamed. I don't feel ashamed now because I talk to my husband. I don't make a ruckus. My husband said, "If a woman offers to have sex with me, I won't accept. I can control myself now." I have one child who always has condoms in his pocket. When I asked him, "Where did you get those condoms?" He said, "I took them from a child who was playing with them." I said, "Good because I know you use them."

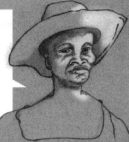

The role-play helped me learn how to think. We got to talk about what we think. I learned how to talk to my husband. I saw the pictures so I know it's true. I make my husband put condoms in his pocket. I learned how to give him advice. All the stories are good because they're the truth. He hears me because he used to go out at 1 a.m. and come home at 4 a.m. Now he goes out at 1 a.m. and comes back at 2 a.m. Our life changed.

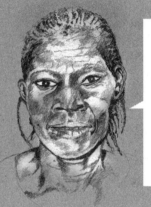

This program gave me light. I have a vagabond. I tell him about Toma and Sentana. What I say is how we said it in the center . . . how to have sex and how to ask him if he had sex with other women. I ask him many questions. When he gets mad, he says, "What kind of questions are these?" I ask him if he uses condoms. He asks me why I ask him this question. I ask him if he has other women. Before, I wouldn't ask him questions. I'd just go to sleep. If he says "yes" he's going to some woman's house, I tell him that if he gets a disease, he will be humiliated. I ask him if he uses anything. Sometimes he laughs, but I know he has condoms in his pocket now. Sometimes he says, "Those meetings you go to are spoiling you." He's changed. After I started talking to him, he started giving me money.

The stories gave me problems because I have a husband who doesn't protect himself. So when I went through the program, I thought, "I can get AIDS too." When I talk, he never listens to me. I talk to his friends. They talk to him but he says I tell lies about him. Now I refuse sex with him without condoms. He talked to the supervisor. He said he knows things from the books now. He told me, "There are thing that I'm sure I could talk to you about, but you think you know more than me now."

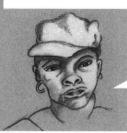

My friend asked me where I found this information. After the program, he asked me to have sex with him. I asked him to get a blood test. He hasn't done it. I won't have sex with him.

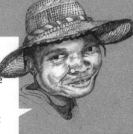

When I saw the books, I began to believe AIDS is real. My husband doesn't believe AIDS is real. He didn't see the stories—so he thinks I'm giving him lies. He says, "You're telling me these things to scare me." I tell him about Toma and Sentana. I tell him to use condoms when we have sex, but he doesn't want to use them. Then I refuse to have sex . . . so we have arguments. We haven't done it very often. The truth is he doesn't know how to use a condom. If the children weren't here, he would force me. He doesn't believe me, but the children have confidence in what I tell them.

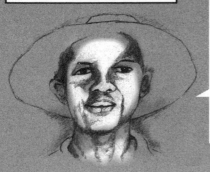

I shared what I learned with friends. If I didn't participate in this program, I wouldn't have knowledge to share. I would be afraid of people with AIDS. We will do whatever you ask us to continue this program. I know a man can refuse sex and a woman can too. There is a story that talks about that. If my wife has a problem, she can say "no" in the same way I can tell my wife what I feel. My wife should talk to me freely. I am responsible for my wife and she is responsible for me. If a woman asks me for something, I should not think about sex in return. If a woman asks me for money because she wants to have sex with me, I can agree to that.

I really loved the story about Toma and Sentana . . . that's why I talk to my wife about it because we have a lot of children and this could happen to me. Now I know what to do. . . . After I was in this program, a friend told me he had sex and pus was coming out of his penis. He is really shy. The doctor gave him an injection. I asked him, "The person who you go the disease from, did you tell her?" He said, "No, I was too ashamed." I told him, "You don't have to be ashamed because you could have given it to her or she could have given it to you . . . you need to prevent this from happening again." I don't know if he talked to her.

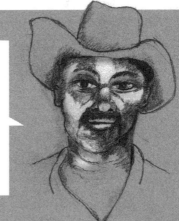

If you are out for a long time, your wife feels she needs to have sex, the husband needs to come back and share love with his wife— even if the husband sends his wife money. If a man doesn't get love from his wife, he will go to another woman. Communication is important . . . otherwise everyone does what he wants. I learned this in the program. It made my brain work better when I saw the pictures.

I talk to my wife about Toma. It really touched me. I asked my wife, "If I leave the house for a long time when I come back, you can ask me if I had sex with other women." I tell her we need to have good communication to avoid problems. She might be ashamed to say she had sexual relations with someone else if I asked her. I tell her, "If you don't talk, I won't know what's on your mind."

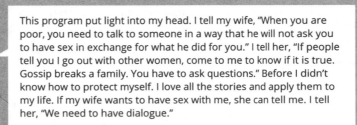

This program put light into my head. I tell my wife, "When you are poor, you need to talk to someone in a way that he will not ask you to have sex in exchange for what he did for you." I tell her, "If people tell you I go out with other women, come to me to know if it is true. Gossip breaks a family. You have to ask questions." Before I didn't know how to protect myself. I love all the stories and apply them to my life. If my wife wants to have sex with me, she can tell me. I tell her, "We need to have dialogue."

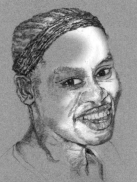

The first day we started the program he didn't change. I started to talk to him. He doesn't act the way he used to. He used to have relationships with other women. I used to have arguments with him. I know how to ask him questions. He knows if he doesn't use condoms, I won't have sex.

She gives me food and doesn't let me leave. We used to fight a lot. We learned that being mean to each other isn't good. If she goes on a trip, when she comes back, I ask her questions. She asks me questions. If my wife says she can't have sex, I agree with her now. Before she would say, she can't have sex and I would say bad things to her. When I wanted to have sex and she didn't, I would force her. After the program, I saw this violence is not good. If a woman decides she doesn't want to do something, her husband should let her think freely. It's normal. The man shouldn't think if his wife refuses, she doesn't love him.

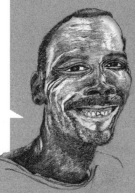

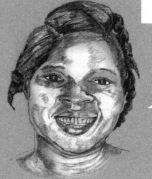

My husband has made a lot of corrections. This program taught him how to listen . . . how to be with me. Before the baby would cry and he would never pick it up. Sometimes he would go to church and just leave me. Now he takes the baby and goes ahead to church so that I can get ready. This program showed him the need to share. Now when he goes out, he always tells me where he's going. He tells me, "When you don't talk with your wife, you don't know what she thinks, what makes her happy or unhappy." There are a lot of people who regret they didn't join this program . . . will it continue?

He told me his group talks about whether men should beat women. If one day a person feels like doing something that's not good, that person will remember what they learned in this program and they will not do it. Before we used to have arguments. There is a change in the way we have sex. When we sleep together, we talk and touch each other. We fight less. Before, we didn't sleep together in the same bed. Since the program, we lie in the same bed and we reconcile. If you don't have understanding, even if you have money, you will have problems. He used to tell me there is no such thing as AIDS. Now he believes me. I feel very proud.

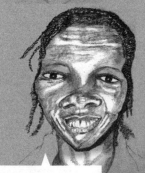

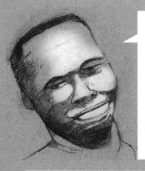

We talk about Toma and Sentana. It's a great example. After hearing the story, it won't happen to us because the training is so good. Now we talk and we try to understand each other. My wife told me that she doesn't feel comfortable using condoms. I know I can be faithful. I ask myself, "Can I keep from going to other women?" I tell her I can, but whenever I feel that I can't resist, I tell her I will use a condom. We feel more prudent. I feel more assured. I can live better than before.

Since I've been talking to him, he said he's not going to have any more relationships with other women. He used to treat me badly. This program is really good for me because if it wasn't for what I learned, I wouldn't have known what to tell him. I feel more confidence in myself.

Our relationship is better. He talks to me now. Life has become better. He knows how to speak to me to put me at ease because he found a person who can explain these things to him. When he has something, he doesn't regret giving it to me.

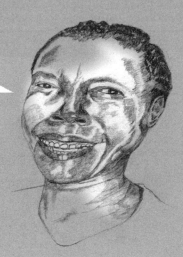

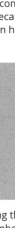

If he is really following the lessons he told me, he will stop doing bad things. He will remember what he talked about in the program and he won't do it.

He told me he learned how to use condoms and how to avoid AIDS. He showed me how to people put condoms on . . . before, my husband didn't know how to use a condom. He talked to me about the stories. What he learned in the program makes him have more love for me. He caresses me more. Before he didn't know what to do to stop having children. I noticed he talks another way now . . . about subjects he didn't talk about before. We are closer than we used to be.

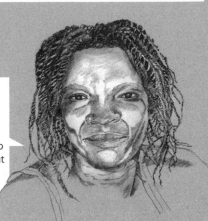

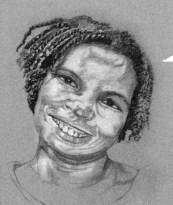

I'm his sister. He talks more to me now and he seems more attached to his children. He is my counselor. He has more knowledge now. His wife told me that he changed the way her talks to her. He showed his wife the books and she told me she likes this program so much. He told me before he didn't know how to use a condom but now he does. Sometimes he says, "I'm in a hurry now because I'm going to the learning center this afternoon. We'll talk later."

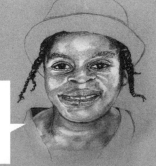

When I used to talk to him, he used to answer me arrogantly. Now he doesn't act like this. He used to have fun with other women . . . he doesn't do that anymore. Before I would wake up in the morning and ask him for money and he wouldn't have any. I knew someone else was profiting from what I was supposed to receive. He says he doesn't care about that anymore.

I don't hit her but sometimes what I say makes her react to me. She told me the stories. She told me what will happen if I sleep with other women . . . I've almost stopped but not yet. She doesn't want me to catch a disease. She's learned to ask me about sex—all the time now. Sometimes she puts her arms around me, and talks to me in a nice way. She used to talk to me in a rough way. I've noticed a change in her.

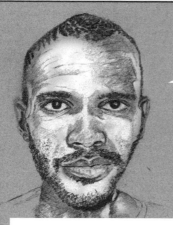

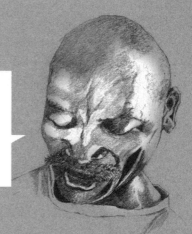

Sometimes she asks me to wear a condom and I say, "No, I don't want to." She said, "I participated in a program and I know how men are living on the outside. I don't work where you work. So I don't know if you met someone outside or not." She didn't used to tell me things like that. She's changed. My wife is more confident now. I know who I am—if I don't protect myself, I'll be a roach in front of a hen. If I do, I'll be a roach inside a bottle.

My wife talks about things she didn't talk about before. Now, she talks to me about sex with condoms. I ask her questions and she talks.

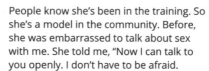

People know she's been in the training. So she's a model in the community. Before, she was embarrassed to talk about sex with me. She told me, "Now I can talk to you openly. I don't have to be afraid.

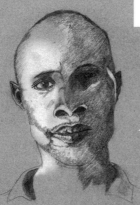

She talked to me how jealousy can break up a family. I do my best to listen to her. When she came from the program, she told me, "I can raise my daughters correctly, but you need to help me raise my sons." She is raising one of my children and five of her children from another man. I talk to her children now . . . especially the sons.

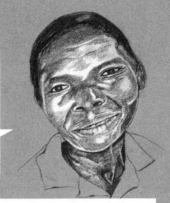

After I leave the center and go home, I sit down with my children and tell them what I learned. Sometimes I lie down in my bed and everyone gathers around me. Sometimes we use candles. I hold the book and I ask them what they see in the pictures—the way the monitor explained it to us. If I don't have a book, I tell them the stories. I don't make the children scared to talk to me because they told me if you make the children scared to talk to you, they will never tell you when they have a problem.

Before I didn't know how to talk to them, but now I talk to my children. Like I have a daughter who is really pretty and men want to be with her. I tell her to protect herself because there are men who are sick who will give her 10 *gourdes* to be with her. I tell her to come to me if you need the money and I'll give it to you.

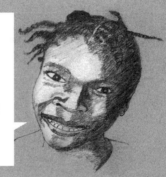

I recently talked to my two daughters about how they can use condoms if they ever they want to have a relationship with a man and don't want to become pregnant. I know that someday they will not be able to resist. Before I didn't share anything with them. Now I talk to them about AIDS. I tell them not to be afraid of someone with it. You know normally parents and children are ashamed to talk like this. Now my children are very happy when I talk to them.

Before I never talked to my mother about sexual things. My mother told me a story about a girl who was infected by her boyfriend. Our relationship has changed. She knows about AIDS and when she comes home from the program, she talks and explains things to us. I'm happier because she teaches us things we don't learn in school. In school when we are talking about sex, we joke. But at home, I can talk with my mother and I understand things better.

Before she started the program, she was always busy. But now, after she started the program, she sits down with us every weekend and talks to us about what she learned. When we leave the house now, she asks us where we are going. She asked me to ask my boyfriend if he is in love with someone else. She always leaves whatever she is doing to go to the program. She teaches us how to take precautions and told us about blood tests.

I have a good opinion of my mother because she has become better. She is more confident. She speaks better. When we are not working, she tells us stories. Sometimes it seems like she talks about AIDS everyday. She talked to me about my body—how my vagina looks on a piece of paper and how many holes I have. She is easier to talk to now.

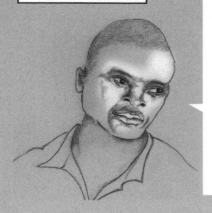

The key was dialogue. When you converse, you can express happiness, sadness, anger, and this allows people to express themselves and share their ideas. These methods show you that you don't have to impose something on someone. When I work with non-literate people, if I tell them whatever they say is not good, they will be afraid of me. Now when I show them I am learning from them, they give more and they are ready to receive as well. This program shows you how to listen. Many health programs use information, condoms, how you get AIDS, but this one uses stories. The participants were really happy. They wanted to go over the stories again and again. They laughed a lot. The stories and pictures allow people to see something real—what is really happening in their lives. The methods allow people to discover themselves. They loved the methods because they made people think about reality. This is the way to break the silence.

One thing that really surprised me was the way participants gained so much confidence to talk about sexual subjects. Now they're not ashamed to talk. You don't see results very often here. In the role-play, they decided roles, laughed, shared stories—this kind of situation is very new here. They wanted to come to the program. They went home to talk with their partners. The stories spoke to them because these were the stories of their lives. All of this gave them confidence to speak.

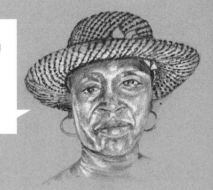

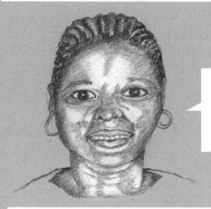

One participant's husband disagreed about using condoms. He said that condoms don't give pleasure. Then I taught her how to use condoms. Afterwards her husband came up to me and said, "Oh, I congratulate you. My wife wanted me to use a condom but I didn't want to because I didn't know how to use it, but now I do."

The pictures are very expressive. They make people think about reality. When you ask questions about what they see in the pictures, they express themselves. They talk about their views. It allows everyone to talk. Everyone can have a personal view about something. By these women telling stories, they are freeing themselves. It doesn't have to be personal, but at the same time it often is.

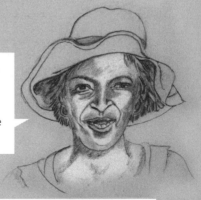

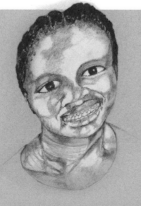

There is a total change. I noticed confidence in their sexual relations and in their relations with some people who are sick in their community. One man told me his sexual relationship is better because he can talk about sex and condoms and use them when he wants to. In the past he said he never talked about these things with his wife. I wanted to talk to a participant. So I told her husband to tell his wife I would be waiting for her that afternoon. He said, "Yes . . . of course." He used to beat his wife and I can see he and his wife are different with each other now.

Conclusion

Participants were expectant because they were being educated. They believed "An educated person is somebody." Though most participants could not read or write, this program contained books and written stories. Participants gained confidence and respect from others because of their newfound knowledge. They said things like:

> *When my family and friends see me go out in the afternoon, they know I don't waste my time. I feel I know more than they do. I feel proud.*

> *When a woman has an argument with her husband, I can tell her how to talk to him now. Now people respect me more because they know I know more than they do.*

> *If someone doesn't believe me, he has to respect me because I'm the one training him.*

> *Once people knew I had a certificate, they would come and ask me questions.*

Credibility was central to whether participants were willing to talk to others about what they learned and about whether others were interested in what they had to say. With books in hand, participants, whether literate or not, showed people they had something valuable to tell them.

In this example of *Toma and Sentana*, the first narrative in the Haitian HIV/ AIDS program, I have given the reader a sense of the process of narrative practice in the creation, practice, and impact of one story. Ironically, before the story of *Toma and Sentana* was introduced, a middle-class Haitian who had been living in Washington, DC, for twelve years read this story and advised us to take it out of the program. He said that Haitians would take offense. Because this story was based on the initial research, we kept it in. As it turned out, *Toma and Sentana* became the most popular story. *Toma and Sentana* became a vanguard for the entire program so that participants started jokingly calling each other Toma or Sentana, drawing attention to their camaraderie. Rather than feeling insulted, people felt pride in this story of their lives.

Gatekeepers from the educated middle classes are often obstacles to effective sexual health education. Whenever I began a project I heard things like "Girls are virgins until they marry" or "No one will talk to you about sex"—all of which proved incorrect. Gatekeepers live by assumption. They arrive at their perceptions as uninformed upholders (though not necessarily followers) of public morality. To acknowledge that poverty is not a moral failing is to abandon the righteousness of privilege: "If they could only be like us . . . all else will follow." This conceals a morality born out of position and power, not one out of honesty and understanding. As one Haitian peasant said, "The rich cannot listen to us because if they did, they would have to see us as people."

In 2008 I returned to Haiti to evaluate the children's rights program. I decided to find people who had participated in the sexual and reproductive health program in 2003. I wanted to find out what they remembered and what had taken hold. In a market, I met a group of Fonkoze women and showed them the books to jog their memories. This is what they said: "Oh, yes, I remember that program! [She laughs]. We talked a lot about sex. I loved this program. I talked with my children about it. We can't always stop men from doing these things but we learned to talk. It was fun . . . we laughed and laughed. Um . . . yes . . . I remember . . . we would like to do this program again."

Another woman added, "This program made me aware of things . . . things I could not say before. It gave me strength. My relationships with people changed . . . I changed. I no longer felt my husband could be anyway he wants. We talk more. I have more to say and I say it. I remember that story of *Toma and Sentana*."

A third woman said, "Everyone remembers that story. It was about our lives. This was a beautiful program for us."

Today the HIV/AIDS, sexual and reproductive health, children's rights, and environment programs are part of Fonkoze's education strategy. The programs under the umbrella *Education is a Conversation: I Want to Live! We Want to Live! Don't You*, have reached thousands of Fonkoze members, their families, and the communities in which they reside.

Narrative practice motivated people to speak in the face of past shame rather than be imprisoned by it. In the process of this practice people reflected and conversed, which encouraged them to decide what was possible and how to achieve it. I would be naïve if not dishonest to claim that this program completely transformed Haitian interactions so that everyone who went through a program was able to reduce his or her risk of HIV infection and/or other vulnerabilities. However, I found a willingness of participants to talk about things that they had not been able to talk about before. Above all, people gained courage to speak. This is one strength of narrative practice—it can collectively reconfigure a public narrative. What matters is that participants changed their conversations because they wanted to live better and because they wanted others in their families and communities to live better as well.

7 | Reflections

I have heard stories about how narrative practice transformed people's conversations and their lives. I have also heard about people who wanted to change their lives and tried but could not accomplish the change they wanted.

Narrative Disappearance and Recovery in the Person of Manuela

Though narrative practice is not therapeutic in the Western sense, in this brief picture of Manuela, I will describe how an individual repaired herself and changed her relations with others after being in a program.

The Latino program in Los Angeles included undocumented Latino men and women who worked primarily as day laborers and domestics. At that time, the HIV rate was increasing among Latinas in the US, second only to the rate among African American women. The Latino program focused on sexual and reproductive health and focused on HIV prevention and AIDS.

Manuela was a peer educator in the Latino program who volunteered at the Mar Vista Gardens Community Center. She also lived in Mar Vista Gardens, a huge, gated community of barrack-like apartments. Over two thousand people lived in Mar Vista, which was notorious for gangs, drugs, and violence. Manuela spoke a little English, but not enough for me to talk to her without a translator. She had lived in America as an undocumented immigrant for over twenty years. Manuela was not just overweight. Her figure ballooned out into mounds of flesh upon flesh. Her head seemed to balance precariously on top, with her small face exuding an expression of fatigue and overuse. Allowing momentum and gravity to assist, Manuela swayed from side to side as she tried to propel herself forward. In the beginning, she hardly radiated the enthusiasm one would have hoped for from a peer educator. When I first met her, she avoided eye contact with me. Her voice was a bare whisper. However, she wanted to be a facilitator. She came to the training regularly.

As I got to know Manuela, I learned about her life. When she was very young, a man wanted to marry her, but then two men raped her. After that, her father made her marry one of the rapists, her current husband. "During my marriage, he continued to rape me," she said. "He was perpetually drunk . . . he had sex with many other women." Manuela told me, "I want to pass over this resentment and not hate my husband all the time. Sometimes when I make him soup, if he doesn't like it, he throws it at me."

Her low opinion of herself was apparent in everything about Manuela, what she said and what she did. During the training when she practiced leading a discussion, her voice was colorless. However, Manuela was compassionate and nonjudgmental, and I noticed this when, at the training, she befriended Maria, a transgender Latino sex worker, while others were uncomfortable with her. I was not sure Manuela could read the stories, but with an unassuming attitude, she was pleased to have others read for her. I worried people would drop out of Manuela's group because they would get bored with her lack of affect.

In the end, Manuela's group converted one of the stories into a play, which they performed at the program's certificate ceremony. Her group members talked at length to me about their love for the program under Manuela's leadership.

After two years, when I was leaving LA, I made a special trip to visit Manuela. She opened the door to her newly acquired office; she got a job in the Mar Vista Gardens Recreation Center as a community organizer. She asked if she could get me something to drink. She still swayed, but her movements seemed less arduous, more purposeful. Manuela smiled and even laughed with me as we tried to communicate in my broken Spanish and her less-fragmented English. What mattered to me was that she was trying to communicate with me over a divide that she had been unable to cross when I first met her. As I was leaving her office, Manuela handed me some plastic flowers on pens, perhaps knowing she would never see me again. She made these for people in her community—one of her gracious acts. At the door she requested the translator's assistance. Manuela looked directly at me and spoke:

> I can help people now. This program changed my life. I feel like a leader now. I can talk about sex and I could never do that before. I have a lot to say . . . things I never said before. Now I say to my husband, "I'm going to give you soup and if you don't like it, you don't have to eat it." I even put condoms in his drawer, and I know he uses them because they disappear. I don't hate as I did before. We live like brother and sister. He is nicer to me. I don't let him treat me badly or talk badly to me. I don't say bad things to him, but I am a changed person and he knows it. . . . Thank you so much.

Manuela walked forward and hugged me. I departed.

Later, in a private conversation with Manuela's two daughters, they confirmed what their mother had said: "Our mother gives us condoms. She talks about sex a lot. Sometimes we laugh and tell her she is nasty, but she is open now. She's really changed. She seems so much happier now than before." Though Manuela most likely will never know this, I owe her a lot. Manuela affirmed what I believe narrative practice can accomplish. She is my evidence.

Marginalization and Shame

By definition, marginalization is the social process of being put or kept in a powerless or unimportant position within a society or group, being on the margins. The social histories of the people in each community where narrative practice was developed fit with this definition of marginality. Poor and marginalized people are subjected to forces of objectification and indifference over which they have no authority. Marginalization historically driven by these forces is effectively outside larger political economies (Farmer 2003).

Impoverished people, without protection, insulation, or resources, are caught in a revolving door of multiple vulnerabilities. How can we characterize their deprivation in ways that could alter this scenario? "Poverty must be seen as the deprivation of basic capabilities rather than merely as inadequate income, which is the standard criterion of the identification of poverty" (Sen 1999:87).

Lacking agency, or the capabilities to effect change, impoverished people often cannot constructively influence their immediate world. Likewise, silence or the inability to converse about shameful subjects takes its toll, particularly among the marginalized: "We are often silent about the ordinary experience of AIDS, the most personal, intimate suffering, just as we are often silent about the most entrenched injustices in the world and how they are perceived by the people who suffer them" (Fassin 2007:277).

In everyday existences, not knowing how to speak or lacking confidence to act is often perceived as the passivity of the poor. I do not believe this is an apt characterization. A question narrative practice tries to answer is: Will people try to change their lives if their vulnerabilities—their sources of shame—are addressed in ways that make sense to them?

Years ago I read about women from impoverished communities in Bangladesh and how they reacted when their children had diarrheal disease. Two groups of women were surveyed to find out why one group brought their children to a clinic before the child fell deathly ill while the other group waited too long and their children sometimes died of dehydration. When interviewed, the two groups of women had similar knowledge and understanding of diarrheal disease. However, the group of women who took their children to a clinic before they became severely dehydrated had attended a few years of elementary school and the other group had never attended school. The former saw themselves as modern women, because of their education, and felt comfortable going to a clinic and conversing with the staff there. The others who failed to act lacked confidence in a clinical setting. When I read this study, I was intrigued by how the self-confidence of the mother made the difference as to whether a child thrived or died rather than knowledge, which played a lesser role.

What was missing for these Bangladeshi women who failed to bring their sick children to a clinic, or in Manuela who was initially so passive? The education these women lacked was not more knowledge per se, but education that would enhance their confidence and competence to act. Forces of marginalization caused inaction for the women of Bangladesh and for Manuela because their anticipation of shame overrode possibilities for taking action for themselves and their children.

Manuela's cumulative experiences of personal abuse together with her marginalization as an undocumented worker led to narrative disappearance (her inability to speak). Her shame was evident in her physical appearance and in her absence of emotional expression. Becoming a peer educator, talking about the narratives, and engaging women in conversations about abuse led to Manuela's newfound courage. She acknowledged shame and gained pride from her engagement with others.

Emotional and Cultural Resonance

Participants talked about how the stories were their own, how they saw themselves in the story characters, and how everything in the stories was true—"everyone can find a story that they have lived." However, in Northern Uganda, I worried that perhaps the stories in the program were too morose considering participants' experiences of war. I decided to add a few comic stories based on Northern Ugandan folk heroes. I met a faculty member at Makerere University in Kampala who was from Northern Uganda and had collected folk tales there. I was surprised to see that many were similar to the Uncle Remus stories in the United States. I wrote five folktales, with characters that mirrored the qualities of Northern Uganda folk heroes, but with comic plots that reflected the issues in the program. When I field-tested the program, I was worried that participants might think the Hare stories were offensive, not funny.

Here are excerpts of one folktale entitled *Hare Boozes*. In this story Hare asks his wife for food but she refuses because he is always drinking with his friends and thus failing to support his family (fig. 7.1).

In Figure 7.2, Hare's wife says, "Oh, so you think I am a useless dog that you brought here to suffer? I will not feed your anus! Feed it yourself!"

Meanwhile we see Hare giving food to his girlfriend (not shown). Then Hare's wife tells him he should leave because her mother is coming soon and she must

Figure 7.1

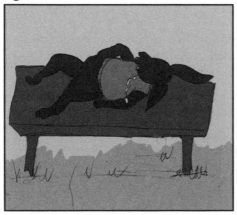

Figure 7.2

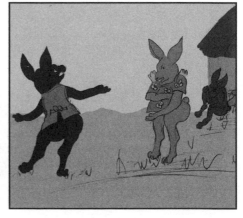

Figure 7.3

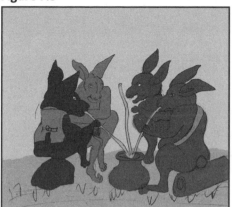

Figure 7.4

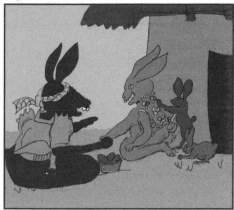

Figure 7.5

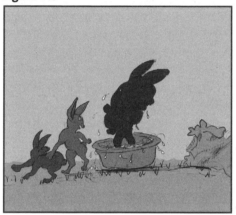

prepare food for her. Hare goes to his drinking friends and discusses his predicament (fig. 7.3). Soon Hare's mother-in-law arrives and Hare's wife tells her mother about her problems with Hare (fig. 7.4):

Hare's wife: My husband wants to kill me. I want to pack my things and go. Mother, can we give him back his ugly cow?

Hare's mother-in-law: Why Hare is a very fine man. If you leave Mr. Hare, your children will suffer. Another woman cannot care for children who are not hers. Um . . . your food is so tasty dear. So tasty!

Hare's wife tells her children to prepare a bath for their grandmother (not shown). Hare's mother-in-law says that she does not need a bath but her daughter insists that she does. While the children are washing their grandmother's back, the grandmother tells them she can wash herself but the children insist. As the children wash her, they notice something unusual about their grandmother (fig. 7.5):

They sound the alarm: Mother! Mother! Grandmother has an animal thing
    between her legs!

In Figure 7.6, Hare's wife realizes that Hare has disguised himself as her mother. Hare's wife goes to the clan. They tell Hare he should stop boozing and start fulfilling his wife's needs. In Figure 7.7, The turtle says, "Really Hare! You must stop wearing *gomesi* [women's dress]. It isn't proper for a man!"

Figure 7.6

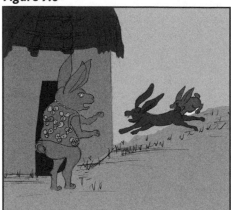

Figure 7.7

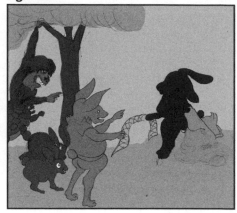

The dialogue in these Hare stories (as in all the stories) was taken from the ethnographic data. References to bride price, an offering of food and a bath to a guest, respect for the elderly, and the idea that a woman cannot take good care of another man's child—these are culturally recognizable to Northern Ugandans.

When I arrived in villages, participants immediately commented on how much they liked the Hare stories—some recounted them word for word. At first I was mystified by this response, but after thinking about it, I realized that the Hare stories made metaphorical sense to the participants. Folk stories use metaphor abundantly to elicit emotion and transformation (Sheub 2006). In the Hare stories, much loved folk heroes were wrestling with serious social problems in comic ways. This use of metaphor resonated with participants.

I also think the Hare stories brought men into the program. They saw in the escapades of Hare that the project was not only for women, which is often men's expectation for sexual and reproductive health programs.

If people respond emotionally to a story, I know that it is culturally credible. People said they laughed uproariously when they heard the stories. The Hare stories have some foul-mouthed discourse. Though few people speak this way, the dialogue was familiar. More so than sadness, humor is often inaccessible to an outsider. I have listened to translations of jokes where I laugh out of politeness but have had no idea what is funny, not knowing if this lack of humor is due to the translation or to something culturally out of reach for me. So I was pleased with the impact of the Hare stories.

Outsiders sometimes view impoverished communities within a mindset of how pathetic they are, ignoring anything that would contradict this belief. Cultural stories carry their own resonance to insiders and within that resonance there is emotional richness. Humor and folk tales are obvious agents of cultural affect. The ribald plots and some of the dialogue in the Hare stories were terrifically lewd but hysterically funny to Northern Ugandans. Ironically one of the foreigners of a supporting organization told me to make sure that visiting donors did not see the Hare tales. Perhaps out of their own propriety, they would have overlooked the joy in these stories and not have understood that, because of this, the program achieved credibility in immeasurable ways.

Qualities of Narrative and of Shame

I will briefly mention an interesting simultaneity inherent in the reparative qualities of narrative and shame in narrative practice. The qualities of shame-filled experiences merge with narrative as the "secret life which each of us lives privately" (Brooks 1984:5). This "secret life" is openly plotted into the composite narratives as the under-story. Each story renders the under-story in textual and visual juxtaposition to the top-story. The structure mirrors the dialectics of shame-filled interactions. Thus, the contradictions within narrative plot and structure not only explicate narrative but also further audience reflection. "Paradox of the self becomes explicitly the paradox of narrative plot as the reader consumes it" (Brooks 1984:52).

Desire is the shaping force of narrative. A psychoanalytic interpretation, inspired by Lacan, describes narrative desire as the following: "irreducible to need, for it is not in principle relation to a real object, independent of subject, rather to a phantasy; it is irreducible to demand, in that it seeks to impose itself without taking account of language and the unconscious of the other, and insists upon being absolutely recognized by the other" (Brooks 1984:55).

Does this not illustrate a driving force of shame—the relentless gaze, which objectifies, stigmatizes, or impersonalizes the other? In one of the narratives, *Rumormongers*, a man's desire to control his wife—based on his fantasy that she should desire only him—leads to violence. In the beginning the husband hears about his wife's flirtations. He demands that his wife recognizes his need, which she cannot satisfy because her husband's *real* need or desire is to control and take revenge. The husband hears his wife has been talking to another man. Others are talking about his wife, thus exposing the husband's inadequacies. "Why," people are saying, "are you not controlling your wife's desires?" In rural Uganda, a "good" married woman is not supposed to publicly reveal desire for any man (including her husband). That the husband has been unfaithful to his wife is of little consequence. The public narrative expects men's infidelities because "he is a man." However, it also expects women's infidelities, though this expectation is based on a husband's economic or sexual failure as motivating factors. Thus the husband tries to repair his shamed self by beating his wife.

Narrative has the reparative capacity not only to evoke memories of desire, but also to reinvent them. Similarly, during narrative practice, participants collectively created narrative endings—retrieving past provocations of shame, while reconfiguring alternative ones. The participants in practice did not renounce past frustrated desires, but they reinterpreted these desires in a revised public narrative.

This collective reconstruction made reasonable sense. As story characters negotiated, the audience in turn renegotiated such transactions in their lives and thus,
in a sense, re-transacted a personal and re-storied resolution. People, like the story
characters, desired something better for themselves. However, what was unrealiz-
able for story characters became realizable for participants.

No one person was the author of the changed public narrative because it was
created collectively. Participants gave testimonials and acted as witnesses; they became actors and spectators. No one person was the producer of a revised public
narrative: "In a web of human relationships . . . the stories, the results of action
and speech, reveal an agent, but this agent is not an author or producer. Somebody
began it and there is a subject in the twofold sense of the word, namely, its actor
and sufferer, but nobody is its author" (Arendt 1958:184).

Participants came to new understandings of themselves with and in the presence of others. Dialogue inspired by the composite narrative created new discourses and meanings. "Dialogue represents a centerless and reversible structure,
engendering an interminable process of analysis and interpretation, a dynamics of
the transference in which the reader is solicited not only to understand the story,
but to complete it: to make it fuller, richer, more powerfully ordered, and therefore, more hermeneutic" (Brooks 1984:260).

In reference to the Ugandan story *Rumormongering*, participants told me that
because of this story, they no longer jumped to conclusions. They conversed with
their partner and others about rumors. They looked at the source of a rumor.
They thought carefully; they became conscious of themselves and more aware of
others regarding the causes and consequences of rumormongering. I was told this
by women and men who had directly experienced or witnessed the violent consequences of rumors.

The Emergence of Collective Change

The significance of an act of solidarity is described in Primo Levi's memory of a
political prisoner who was able to switch prisoner's registration numbers to con-
demn some to death and prevent others from dying. By switching the numbers of
cruel prisoner guards (so they were put to death) with prisoners who were being
abused, this political prisoner was in solidarity with the latter. In Levi's mind this
prisoner was beyond the reach of shame (Levi 1989:74). I bring up this point because
in my observations of marginalized people, there is at times a debilitating absence
of moral solidarity. People in impoverished communities have been pejoratively
likened to crabs in a basket—fighting each other for sparse, diminishing resources.
They cannot openly address their vulnerabilities because these are perpetuated by
influences outside their immediate world like those of structural violence (Farmer
2003). Some turn to local clandestine practices, such as potions and incantations,
which are believed to reduce their vulnerabilities (Farmer 2006; Ashforth 2004).
These practices point to the cause, a witch for example, of intangible nefarious

forces, and inspire fear of those perceived responsible (like someone suspected of being HIV positive). Hidden practices sustain a pervasive state of marginality and deter solidarity. Narrative practice led to solidarity because it engendered a praxis of shame, publicly and collectively.

In the following I will describe this praxis in examples of empathetic, re-integrative, and stigmatizing shame. Each participant in these three different manifestations acknowledges shame through narrative practice, and these acknowledgements were reparative for them. However, narrative practice led to different ways that shame was experienced, and as a consequence, different outcomes.

Empathetic Shame

Evaluation interviews from the Haitian children's rights program focused on the treatment of children in general as well as on children in *restavek*. For a 'child in *restavek*' it is a move from very poor to less poor. On the pull side, a low income urban or semi-urban family acquires an unpaid servant instead of one for cash. The educated wealthy disdain *restavek* labor in part to show they have resources to hire domestic help. Also, when human rights advocates began to publicize *restavek* labor as child slavery, well-off Haitians lost their taste for it.

On the push side are poor, often large, rural families who send their children to live with an aunt, grandparent, godparent, distant relative (all socially legitimate), or stranger (less socially legitimate) with the expectation that the child will benefit from schooling, clothes, food, and social mobility. The situation of children in servitude is complicated by an extended family system that has the capacity to be life giving and nurturing as well as the opposite, cold and cruel. Parents envision an investment in a child's education as comparable to a bank account for their own and their child's future. Giving one's child away is driven by necessity as much as by hope (Murray and Smucker 2004).

I remember this participant because she was so serious. She was a young woman, slight, soft-spoken but determined. She participated in the program with her mother, and together, they became advocates for children:

> Sometimes my mother and I compare the stories about what we see. Our neighbor has a nephew, and she is treating that nephew like a slave. She is making that child work so hard. The child might be doing something and she interrupts him to do something else before he has finished doing the first thing. He never has time to rest. When the child was eating, before he finished, she would ask the child to do this or that. She used to hit the child with a big stick. So I went to her and told her she should stop treating that child like a slave. I invited her to participate in one of the sessions. She came, and after that, when I talked to her, she tried to make me think it was the child's fault. She has changed because she lives close my house. . . . I see that she is not treating the child the same as she used to. She rarely hits him. When she does, she uses a little stick. This program helps me be a leader for children's rights. I invited several people to our sessions.

Approaching that woman was not an easy thing for me to do because before, though it made me sad seeing the way she treated that child, I had never said anything to her. So by approaching her, I see I am on the right path.

Guilt points toward what has happened to others, shame points to what we are and what we want ourselves to be (Williams 1993:92–93). In the past the daughter and her mother had felt empathy for the plight of mistreated children, but they had done nothing to stop it. During the program, they became aware that they had failed in what they expected of themselves. Engendering empathetic shame, the program recovered who they wanted themselves to be—their better selves. "This program helps people see how it feels to be mistreated as a child. I heard a woman say if the child didn't do something, he wouldn't eat for that day. I talked to her about what I learned. She decided this was not the right way to be."

From narrative practice, participants experienced another's shame and that was shameful for them. They internalized shame in this paradox: the self, who I think I am or want to be, is set against "Who am I in the eyes of others because I am doing nothing?" By speaking out, people gained pride in responding to situations where they saw children being mistreated. For them, shame "promised a return of interest, joy, and connection" (Probyn 2005:xiii).

Re-integrative Shame

I remember another participant in the Haitian children's rights project. This woman was very excited to talk to me. This is what she told me:

I don't know what else to say about this program because I so love it. The program opened my eyes. I am a woman in misery. I gave two of my girls up to stay with their godmother because I couldn't help them like I should. Since I started reading these stories about *restaveks*, I decided to go take my girls back home because that hurt me a lot. What hurt me the most from the books . . . what pushed me the most was when I saw the girl abused. Immediately, I was thinking of my girls. I didn't tell their godmother why I was taking them. I just said to her that I have come to take them to spend a few days with me. But for myself, I already knew why I came to take them. Even if God gave me fifty children, there is not one of them that I would leave with other people! The children who live with other people get mistreated so much. The person who wrote these books does not lie. The stories tell a lot of truths.

What struck me about this woman was the courage it took for her to bring her children home. Perhaps this woman felt ambivalent about giving her daughters away, or the godmother had already shown that she was not kind. Regardless, taking her daughters home was not an easy matter. I did not doubt that this woman, like most parents, loved her children. I think when this woman read, discussed, and acted out the stories, she felt shame in having given her children away. However, this woman also felt shame about her inability to give her children a better life, which initiated her decision to send them away in the first place. What transpired to cause her to retrieve her children? Her collective engagement with others led her to a decision to protect her children from a misery she deemed worse than the misery of poverty.

This woman reflected on her children's lives, and it disturbed her enough to bring her children home. The stories in the Haitian children's rights program address not only the mistreatment of children, but also the subservience of impoverished adults who give their children away to adults who are better off. At the time when she gave her children away, the public narrative did not expose the abuses that her children might suffer living in *restavek*.

In this example of shame's praxis, I see this woman's shameful discovery. It draws on something more innate than empathetic shame, perhaps shame's psychoanalytic signification: in the loss of the other is the loss of the self. This praxis of shame was liberating and re-integrative for this woman because in her retrieval of her children, she retrieved herself.

Stigmatizing Shame

I interviewed a participant who was very much the opposite. The respondent seemed covert and unwilling to talk to me. She would not look at me directly, but kept turning away from me at each question. I sensed that she was lying or trying to evade answering my questions. So I asked the facilitator, who had suggested the interview, why she had wanted me to talk to this woman. This was what the facilitator told me:

> Some people you cannot approach. . . . They don't understand what you tell them. They will take it very badly if you talk to them. But some people really change. Like this woman you were interviewing. Her child misbehaved and what did she do? She took a razor blade and cut the palms of that little boy and cut the bottom of the little boy's feet so he wouldn't walk around. She told him not to go somewhere, but you know how children are. This happened before she was in the program. While she was in the program, some of us talked to her about how she should be treating her children. We told her that when children do something wrong, she should call the children and talk to them. She felt very ashamed and she realized what she did was wrong. She has changed a lot. We usually started the program at five pm, and she was usually here around four pm because she was so interested in the program.

The woman who abused her child wanted others to know she had changed. She demonstrated this by coming early to the sessions, actively participating, and by these actions telling others, "You see, I have changed." Most likely, she will never

cut her child's feet again. But whether she really had changed enough to compre-
hend the cruel thing she did and how her child suffered is a moot point. How can
we know whether she really felt sorry for what she did to her child? The facilitator
told me, "This woman feels ashamed"—but is that because she was found out?

In this woman, we see another manifestation of shame's praxis in stigmatizing
shame. The public narrative changed so that it was no longer acceptable to hit,
cut, or inflict pain on children. Now people in this woman's community might be
watching, commenting on, and noting those who defy this narrative. The group
openly talked to her about what she had done to her child. Shame's praxis in this
woman's case was drawn from the public exposure of a stigmatizing shame, and
after that, this was reparative for her. Just as the stocks, scaffolds, and public hang-
ings of Europe were publicly shaming for people (Gatrell 1994), this woman was
publicly shamed with less severe consequences. After all, consider the power of a
public narrative: if it was shameful *to not* inflict pain on children, would there not
be many willing adherents?

One of the head trainers of the Haitian children's rights program talked to me
about how the program took away fear. In my opinion, the program took away fear
because the public narrative that formerly excused, accepted, or turned a blind eye
to the suffering of children in *restavek* exposed the truth of their abuse. In seeing,
hearing about, and discussing children's plights, participants lost their fear. The
onlookers (the participants) had nowhere else to turn their gaze except on one another. Denial was no longer possible. People desired to repair themselves.

I am reminded of a visit I made to a Northern Thai village in 1992. I see
many nicely constructed, relatively large modern houses with large television an-
tennas protruding from roofs except for one house, which is a shack-like structure without an antenna. My interpreter tells me that the man who lives there
refuses to send/sell his daughters to Bangkok (meaning into prostitution), and
therefore his economic situation is decidedly different from his neighbors. Most
daughters who went to Bangkok send regular remittances to their rural families.
His neighbors urge him to send his daughters to Bangkok, but he holds firm.
They tell him how shameful it is for him to live in such poverty when he has
two perfectly healthy daughters who can change all that. Unbeknownst to them,
in a few years AIDS will change this public narrative in lasting ways. In the
meantime, this father goes against the current public narrative. In this village
the overt wealth of people's homes is out of sync with a backdrop of low-level
farming technology and poor land productivity. About thirty kilometers away
in another village, none of the families send their daughters to Bangkok. In this
other village people live in modest, small houses and shacks.

> When we shame in ways that nurture social bonds, that sustain integration, that
> trigger dialogue in which help is offered. . . . We shame in a way that should pre-
> vent externalized and internalized violence. (Scheff and Retzinger 1991:xiii)

Moral Agency

What is the connection between feelings of shame, narrative practice, and moral agency? Helen Lewis famously described shame and guilt as the moral emotions (1971). Unfortunately, shame has been represented historically as a highly negative emotion (Deonna, Rodogno, and Teroni 2012). A proverbial image of shame is of a person with eyes cast down under the unrelentingly gaze of the other. However, because the shamed one has the capacity to look at what he or she is, shame can be the key to transformation, in returning the gaze or in trying to alter the objectifying gaze of the other. "Shame illuminates our intense attachment to the world, our desire to be connected to others, and the knowledge that, as merely human, we will sometimes fail in our attempts to maintain these connections" (Probyn 2005:14).

Once shame is felt and understood, people will normally try to repair themselves (Tangney and Dearing 2002). If shame goes unacknowledged, violence is sometimes the consequence (Scheff and Retzinger 1991), but acknowledging one's shame might influence resolution for 'the other' in non-reparative ways. For example, to return to *Rumormongering*, the husband in that story, rather than acknowledging his shame, seeks totality in his drive to end the paradox of his suffering. For the husband, beating his wife has a reparative function. In a story of Indian women 'coolies' working on sugar cane plantations outside of India in the 1800s, Indian men felt shamed because their women were openly changing partners if a better economic or sexual option came along. Nevertheless, while many Indian men admitted their humiliation, this did not stop them from brutalizing and murdering Indian women in unprecedented ways and numbers (Bahadur 2014). The goal of the one who experiences a loss of self (in his or her loss of the other) is to close the gap, to heal himself or herself, but not necessarily to heal the other. Whom is the shamed person repairing, in what context and why, and to what consequence?

Because public narratives express ways people choose to repair themselves, they give credence, if not a sanctioning guide, to one's private actions. If the reparation of one's shame requires one to punish others, then how is the moral good in that community configured? If the reparation of one's shame requires dialogue with the intention of forgiveness of others, then how is the moral good in that community configured?

Participants publicly discussed the story *Rumormongering*, knowing full well that rumors were a source of violence in their communities. They spoke about how people within their communities could reduce the causes and consequences of rumors. Situated within their community, in a process of collective reparation, people reinterpreted shame and vulnerability. In essence, they revised the public narrative: "the projection of the criticizing agency can be carried out to constructive ends. The person projects it on to, or in to, the environment in order . . . to find a measure of shared agreement with friends and acquaintances" (Wollheim 1999:219).

One can see a relationship between shame and moral agency in the Truth and Reconciliation Commissions and in the writings of John Braithwaite (1989, 2002) about restorative justice. Truth and Reconciliation Commissions seek restorative justice through reconciliation rather than through punishment. Restorative justice is a form of public reconciliation between perpetrators and victims. According to Braithwaite, restorative justice is:

> a process where all stakeholders affected by an injustice have an opportunity to discuss how they have been affected by the injustice and to decide what should be done to repair the harm. With crime, restorative justice is about the idea that because crime hurts, justice should heal. It follows that conversations with those who have been hurt and with those who have inflicted the harm must be central to the process. (Braithwaite 2004:28)

Similar to narrative practice, restorative justice entails a public recognition of a tormenting shame as a basis for reparation. An underlying tenet of both is that acknowledged shame can repair broken bonds and unacknowledged shame can aggravate disagreement and lead to rage and escalating conflict (Scheff and Retzinger 1991:167–68). In a process of reparation, dialogue is fundamental to both narrative practice and restorative justice.

Narrative practice and restorative justice take the view that injustices are not caused by evil as much as by power, indifference, ignorance, lack of public will, the discomfort of changing what one is used to, or lack of understanding of the wrongs being done to others. In the Truth and Reconciliation process in South Africa, some people asked for forgiveness, having been unaware of the hurt they had caused others (Scheper-Hughes 2007). In narrative practice I heard the same thing: people talked about the shame they felt from having caused harm to others. They explained that they were unaware of how another person felt or of how their actions were a source of another person's pain. As one man said about abusing his wife: "I feel so shameful and painful because I really felt I shouldn't have done that. There are things in the program that really touched me . . . things I didn't understand before. I really had shame and thought about it because we had no peace in my home . . . because of what I did."

While restorative justice shares aspects with narrative practice, there are differences in their nature, scale, process, and intent. Narrative practice is localized at the community level and seeks to change social and intimate interactions through composite narratives and a practice. The intent is reparation on the small scale of everyday personal interactions.

Reparation in narrative practice is not necessarily perceived as reconciliation between definitive offenders and victims. Narrative practice avoids labels. While people talk about shameful subjects in narrative practice, the person who provokes shame is not directly exposed and does not publicly talk to the person who has been shamed. Dimensions of power in narrative practice are not so clear-cut between the one who shames another and the one who is shamed. Acts of reparation are seen as commonplace interactions that have the potential to heal or hurt because a shamed person will try to heal her or himself.

Reparation of the self is located in unavoidable, constant relations with others. Therefore, narrative practice seeks repair, not through public apology and community service in place of punishment, but through everyday experiences of reparative (often private) conversations.

Social Justice

Bertolt Brecht poignantly states the power of this understanding: "the compassion of the oppressed / for the oppressed is indispensable. / It is the world's only hope" (1997:328). Narrative practice inspires collective actions for social justice. According to Bourdieu, one's relation to power determines what is possible (1990:64). We can see how Haitians transformed these relations. The Haitian children's rights program was implemented in IDP camps that were set up after the earthquake in 2010. Facilitators were trained in the narratives and their methodologies. As a consequence of the children's rights learning groups, camp communities elected Child Protection Committees. These committees served as watchdog groups to uncover child abuse and to link incidents of mistreatment of children in *restavek* with social service agencies in order to find help for these children. Groups of survivors of mistreatment (former *restaveks*) formed support groups. International NGOs requested their staff be trained in the narratives and methodologies. The children's rights program in Haiti expanded conversations about children in servitude from the community to the national level. The solidarity achieved in learning groups extended to acts of collective responsibility, and thousands have benefitted. Today there is an impending possibility that the Haitian government might officially take a stronger stand to officially eradicate the practice of child servitude altogether.

All this leads me to the question of whether poor people care about rights. Amartya Sen states that a state of justice often moves people (1999). Within the Haitian children's rights program, people sought justice because they were emotionally touched enough to respond to the social shame and silence surrounding the mistreatment of children. People acquire voice through consciousness-raising when it is a social process involving public interactions (Sen 1999). Acquiring voice—the confidence and competence to speak—is a means of overcoming social injustice and invisibility. Because of the children's rights program, people made more just decisions regarding the treatment of children. They arrived at these decisions because public narratives were not only openly exposing the mistreatment of children, but also suggesting that people could do something about it.

The narratives are not necessarily illuminating problems so much as giving public voice to hidden (though known) ones. In most communities, neighbors know who is being abused, who is HIV infected, who is suffering. However, few will speak out or help because the underlying issues are circumscribed by feelings of shame and fear. Some believe it is not their business, or they do not want to offend their neighbor or cause trouble, or they do not know what to say or do. A shamed person is stigmatized, and few will risk talking to or helping someone so labeled. Any action outside the norm could bring shame for the person who initiated this action. Few will risk this.

According to Walter Benjamin, a story possesses moral power because it makes it possible to bring others into our lives (in Lara 2007:89). The moral power of narrative practice brought people into each other's lives in ways that made them want to think better of themselves and others, and improve how others saw them. The result was, as this woman simply stated, "We talked about the stories and people felt ashamed of their behavior . . . starting with me. I used to hit children a lot. I used to humiliate them. Neighbors would listen and hear me. I don't do this anymore. I want to be a better person, so that people can say good things about me."

Acts of Generosity and Pride

Narrative practice is transformative because it inspires simple acts of generosity and of pride. I believe healthy communities (not necessarily wealthy ones) thrive out of these acts. When I lived in rural areas in the developing world for any extended period of time, my neighbors, or anyone I visited, would give me something they valued to show their appreciation.

In Ethiopia I remember visiting the home of one of my students whose family was very poor. The family offered me a glass of coffee, half of which was butter. For guests or celebrations, Ethiopians add a small amount of butter to coffee, but this amount far exceeded the imaginable—three cups or at least six month's supply for this family. I felt certain that if I drank it, I would die on the spot. But when I tried to refuse, I sensed my host's deep embarrassment. More recently in Uganda, in 2012, I visited a man and his two wives. He felt that the program transformed his relationships with his wives and their relationship with each other. As I left his household, he gave me two live chickens. I was on a motorbike. Carrying these two bound chickens would be a struggle. Though they had a lively flock, chicken was this family's only source of meat for a household of twelve. I told them that I could not eat a chicken that I had developed a friendship with, and I had already become familiar with this chicken. The family laughed, probably thinking, "She's crazy." I understand that as a "rich" outsider, I am allowed a long rope of tolerance far beyond the normally acceptable. I ended up with one chicken and a jar of shea butter.

I have witnessed acts of generosity that would be difficult to understand, or of little matter to an outsider, and yet these have deep cultural affinities. A participant reflected on the significance of acts of generosity because of the Uganda program:

> We never shared food or drank in one pot with someone outside. This can lead to loss of life. But God created a way. . . . All of us met in the training as a group

and we were able to settle our issues and right now as I talk, we can share food and drink from one pot, and we can sit together and talk. They have even given me the garden so I can dig freely. . . . Right now, they no longer hate me and we are free.

Without benevolence, people starve, not for want of food but for want of community. In the presence of acts of generosity communities thrive or, in their absence, disintegrate.

When well-off and well-intentioned outsiders arrive in an impoverished community and flood people with money and gifts that are dramatically outside the values or capabilities of that community, what does this do? In essence, this might be stealing an essential aspect of any healthy community: its intrinsic generosity. The power of a wrong view is measured by the power of a gift experienced by those who are powerless to reciprocate. The wrong view gains credence for the ones who receive when this wrong view becomes their own view of themselves. When receivers absorb a wrong view, communities break down or cease to value their own acts of generosity. "In order for symbolic power domination to be set up, the dominated have to share with the dominant schemes of perception and appreciation through which they are perceived by them and through which they perceive them; they have to see themselves as they are seen" (Bourdieu 1997:237).

Shame is provoked from an unwanted or wrong view—when we are met with the wrong gaze, the wrong view coming from someone with a certain perception of us that is not who we are. "For the other, even when not an enemy, is regarded only as someone to be seen, not someone (like us) who also sees" (Sontag 2003:72).

Mary Douglas, in her foreword to *The Gift*, comments that "a gift that does nothing to enhance solidarity is a contradiction." She goes on to say that the recipient of a gift that does not enhance solidarity between the giver and the receiver causes the receiver to dislike the giver (1990:vii). Given that the giver has possibly shamed her or him, how could the receiver feel otherwise?

Narrative practice engages people in reciprocity in multiple ways. The sender (the reader or storyteller) and the receiver respond to each other by telling another story or commenting on the story. They are experiencing the gift of a shared story. "An act of generosity to which the receiver should respond by an equal generosity, either in telling another story . . . , or in commenting on the story told . . . by the proof that the gift has been received, that the narrative has made a difference" (Brooks 1994:87).

Oral exchanges like these generate feelings of solidarity. In narrative practice, participants said they had feelings of living shared experiences, which led to feelings of trust and in some cases, forgiveness.

The twenty-three-year war that brutalized Northern Uganda created trauma, distrust, and hatred. Many people lived in refugee camps for years, and during those years the culture of northern Uganda was under assault from many quarters. In the IDP camps, there were numerous instances of rape, abuse, excessive drinking, and vile acts perpetrated by the Lord's Resistance Army (LRA), and by the Ugandan army, which warped the integrity of Northern communal life and caused unrelenting humiliation of the local people (Dolan 2009). Day-to-day life, as it existed before the war, had been severely eroded. In the war's aftermath, many people no longer trusted each other to work together amicably. Returnees (as many as twenty-five thousand), who had been kidnapped by the LRA as children and forced to become soldiers, had been responsible for unspeakable acts of cruelty to local people. People were not readily accepting returnees, but in this, narrative practice helped:

> To me the training has helped so much. People had the spirit of revenge. For example, there are some returnees who were kidnapped as children . . . they were rebels. Whenever the community looks at them, they say, "so-and-so was so terrible . . . he killed my relatives . . . he killed so many people." You feel like taking revenge. You feel like this person should be killed. This training helped release this spirit of revenge and helped people socialize. In our group there were people who returned from the bush. Before people talked about them so much, but since they have been part of the training, people no longer talk about them.

When people say *the bush* they are referring to living in a wild state as child soldiers or as members of the LRA. I interviewed returnees to find out their perceptions. One returnee was a slight man in his twenties, but he looked much older. He told me he had been kidnapped three times when he was in his early teens—the first two times he ran away, but the third time he was unable to leave and lived as a child soldier for five years. This is what he said:

> When I was alone . . . by myself . . . I sometimes had a lot of problems . . . very bad memories. But when I was in the group, you shared, you laughed, and you found solutions to your problems. Those past experiences with the rebels . . . I don't have thoughts about them as much anymore. Because of this program, I know that I should not handle things in a reckless way . . . that can affect my children badly. Because of being in the bush, I dictated to my wife. I realized I was doing harm to my family. Now I share family decisions. I even give my wife money. Also hating one another . . . this program discourages that. People in the program accepted me and listened to my views. I even acted in a role-play!"

Adults felt their culture had been destroyed, and with that, possibilities for productive, collective action. Many young adults who had grown up in the camps rejected farming and preferred going to video halls. The camaraderie of digging groups, a former cornerstone of Acholi culture, had come to an end. "This program is about reconciliation because we've distorted the peace that we initially had . . . the peace that was a part of Acholi culture. We used to eat and dig together, but that was destroyed, so there is a great need to reconcile and reunite in digging groups because when people moved to the camps all that ended."

Narrative practice cultivated acts of generosity toward family, friends, and neighbors, and these acts furthered reconciliation. Keeping in mind the erosion of communality in the aftermath of war, participants in the Uganda program felt transformed because the program helped them to live better with each other:

> Now we share food. We borrow money and hoes. These changes occurred because of this program. It brings people together. This is why there are really community changes. There are good relations among participants. . . . We were able to create new and better friends. We are able to work together in a digging group and when a day is scheduled to move to one of the member's gardens, everyone turns up and works in that garden together. The next day we dig in someone else's gardens. We help each other when there is sickness and take someone to the hospital. We mourn together. It really helps to bring people's minds together to share their problems. We really see how our friends react to certain problems, and that's why there are changes in this community. So however much you hate some people, you learn to share things and ideas . . . you know this program brings humanity and solidarity.

Narrative practice causes transformations when people feel a sense of individual and collective pride. Adults felt pride because they prevented harm to others. In Haiti, Bangladesh, Uganda, and Los Angeles, adults talked about sex, sexuality, and sexual and reproductive health with their children and their children's friends. In these locales it was often culturally prohibitive for parents to talk to their children about sexual health and yet, as a consequence of narrative practice, they did:

> I can tell them a lot of things I could not tell them before. My happiness is from the courage I got to talk to my girls about early marriage and early sex. . . . I didn't do this before. In my culture, it is taboo. I learned if you are not open about sexual intercourse, you might be hurting the future of young ones.

Not surprisingly, most marginalized communities do not have trained counselors or readily available resources to help solve family or community conflicts. Those few who have skills to counsel others cannot meet the myriad number of peoples' counseling needs. Non- or marginally literate participants felt pride in their ability to counsel others, as this woman explained:

> My own sister Florence and her husband had divorced each other because of violence, but when I shared this program with them, the husband traveled all the way from another county . . . and we talked. Since then, they came back together. I have never stepped in a classroom and I don't know what a blackboard looks like, but I

used the skills I learned in this program to get this couple back together. This program helped me build confidence to talk to people.

People felt they were doing something important, saying things like "I am really happy because I feel that I am helping people change." Many who went through a program became ad hoc community counselors and for many, as one old woman enthusiastically said, "This is big work!"

Education Is a Conversation

In the rural areas where I developed most of these programs, communities thrive in busy markets, with hawkers and buyers engaging in constant conversation. This same fluidity of conversation exists everywhere in rural communities. Walking past someone from your neighborhood without acknowledgment is unlikely. Usually there is an exchange, even if only in greetings to the person's family, relatives, neighbors, and a litany of others. These greetings, though not so different than "How are you?" and "I am fine," go far beyond the person in front of you because these are cultures of *we*.

Narrative practice looks to public stories and how they are deeply rooted in us as stories we repeat about ourselves and others. Storytelling is a route to our collective memory and a wellspring of human solidarity. Though the modern world has lost the presence of the traditional storyteller, I often marvel how people at social gatherings repeat what they heard on television or read in newspapers. The primary storyteller today is public media. One step away is the story repeater—the modern day conversational copyist who gains an affirmation of agreement from retelling a media story. In any case, storytelling is ubiquitous, and what is heard in the postmodern world in a secondhand performance is heard firsthand in rural non-technological communities. Stories in every culture are used to galvanize and educate an audience.

However in narrative practice, education through storytelling is much more than a conversation. The process of narrative practice engenders reflexivity as participants become more aware of themselves and their relations with others. The narrative unfolds, and the audience sees how power and powerlessness intertwine, emerge, and disappear in patterned ways. Narrative contradiction causes participants to see how narrative disappearance results from shame and suffering. Narrative transactions occur as story characters negotiate and renegotiate their positions vis-à-vis others. In the story *Widow Inheritance*, when a brother of the dead man refuses to marry the widow, it is the widow who chastises this brother and accuses his wife of bewitching her husband, because she feels shamed at his rejection. While one might see widow inheritance as a brother's choice, there may be more at stake. The stories are not about culpability but rather about how people can address shame-provoking interactions that sustain, increase, or prevent vulnerability.

Narrative practice is a practice of constant human engagement. Learning group members become engaged in retrospection and active dialogue. They share stories and practice conversations. Participants give testimonials as others act as witnesses:

> There was one person in our group who grew up as a *restavek*. She was telling the truth, saying, "If I went to fetch water and I took too much time, the woman beat me. . . . If they woke up in the morning and I hadn't finished washing the dishes, the woman beat me. . . . The children in the household would pinch, poke, and hit me. . . . Whatever happened, I was blamed for everything." When this person was talking, I was thinking, *The child who is living with me, I'm treating her worse than how this woman was treated.* It shocked me to hear about this woman's life.

Participants are asked to give advice to story characters and to choose alternatives for them; participants are asked questions about story characters and then asked what they would do if they were faced with similar predicaments.

This process culminates in a dramatized role-play in which participants must practice negotiation skills in order to solve a real-life problem. This gives the participants ideas for changing similar conversations in their everyday lives. When participants are asked to give commentary on themselves as much as on others, this fosters greater autonomy. Going out into the world and challenging beliefs and practices requires transforming consciousness and building individual self-confidence within collective solidarity:

> The women have been moving with this program to their homes . . . the men respect them because there are so many under this program nearby. Now women have gotten the courage to share their feelings and talk to a man about his behavior and so men, too, are changing.

Narrative practice is inherently a political process in that it draws on memory and tries to reconfigure shame by changing the dialectics of power that gave rise to injustice in the first place. "The most explosive realm of politics is the rupture of the political 'cordon sanitaire' between the hidden and the public transcript" (Scott 1990:19). When an impoverished parent gives his or her child to another family, that parent is subject to the public narrative that the child will have a better life with someone who has money. Publicly acknowledging how children in servitude are abused led to change. Human beings want to close the totality, to repair the self, and to change shame's provocations. We are subjects of shame who can seek repair through acts of violence or, alternatively, through acts of empathy and hope.

In the beginning I stated that this book is an exploration of community narrative practice. You, the readers, are probably not recipients of one of the community narrative practice programs, but are more privileged and educated—possibly students, researchers, program planners, practitioners, or evaluators from industrialized or developing countries. In addition to the importance of cultural context, I have emphasized common ground in our propensities to fear, stigmatize, and blame the 'the other.' Regardless of education, wealth, and status, our capacity to shame and to be shamed is our common ground. For you, the readers, this simple consideration might be as relevant to your work as to the immediacy of daily life.

Narrative practice is not a definitive answer to human vulnerabilities. I hope this book is not seen as a study of impoverished people or as a treatise about how to fix their lives. Rather, the ideas here might be useful in influencing better understanding about, for example, why and how to listen to others. I hope I do not cause harm by exposing stories for public scrutiny that were originally intended for a select audience. I hope narrative practice will provoke questions: How long and in what ways can change from this practice be sustained? How can narrative practice bring change that addresses the lack of or the pollution of resources together with the potential collective strength of community? In what ways could the ideas of narrative practice be usefully applied to other situations with deep-seated under-stories, such as political and corporate corruption?

Education is a Conversation: I Want to Live! We Want to Live! Don't You?, the title of four community narrative practice programs, simply states that we learn in everyday conversation with others. If we share this belief, do we not also share the desire to live more amicably together? In this mutual desire, who among us would not want to learn in conversation with others? Would you not engage in conversation to educate each other if you value other people's desire to have and pursue a just life as you value your own such desire? Community narrative practice transforms what we say, how we listen and speak, what we think and feel, together with how we act to help ourselves live generously with others, a life-sustaining need of all healthy human communities.

References

Abraham, Charles, and Pascal Sheeran
    2007   "The Health Belief Model." In *Predicting Health Behavior*. Mark Connor and Paul Norman, eds. Pp. 28–81. Maidenhead, Berkshire: Open University Press.

Agamben, Giorgio
    1999   *Remnants of Auschwitz*. New York: Zone Books.

Aggleton, Peter
    1996   *Bisexualities and AIDS: International Perspectives*. Bristol, PA: Taylor & Francis.

Arendt, Hannah
    1958   *The Human Condition*. Chicago: The University of Chicago Press.

Aristide, Jean-Bertrand
    2000   *Eyes of the Heart*. Monroe, ME: Common Courage Press.

Aristotle
    1954   *Rhetoric*. New York: Modern Library.

Ashforth, Adams
    2004   "AIDS and Witchcraft in Post-Apartheid South Africa." In *Anthropology at the Margins of the State*. Veena Das and Deborah Poole, eds. Pp. 141–64. Santa Fe, NM: School of American Research Press.

Bahadur, Gaiutra
    2014   *Coolie Woman: The Odyssey of Indenture*. Chicago: The University of Chicago Press.

Bandura, Albert
    1990   "Perceived Self-Efficiency in the Exercise of Control over AIDS Infection." *Evaluation and Program Planning* 13:9–17

Barthes, Roland
    1975   *The Pleasure of the Text*. New York: Farrar, Straus and Giroux.

Benjamin, Walter
    1968   *Illuminations: Essays and Reflections*. New York: Harcourt, Brace & World.

Berger, Peter L., and Thomas Luckmann
    1966   *The Social Construction of Reality: A Treatise on the Sociology of Knowledge*. New York: Anchor Books.

Bourdieu, Pierre
    1990   *The Logic of Practice*. Stanford: Stanford University Press.
    1997   "Marginalia—Some Additional Notes on the Gift." In *The Logic of the Gift: Toward an Ethic of Generosity*. Alan D. Schrift, ed. Pp. 231–45. New York: Routledge.

Braithwaite, John
    1989   *Crime, Shame and Reintegration*. Cambridge: Cambridge University Press.

2002 *Restorative Justice and Responsive Regulation*. Oxford: Oxford University Press.

2004 "Restorative Justice and De-Professionalization, Symposium: Theory of Democratic Professionalism." *The Good Society* 13(1):28–31.

Brecht, Bertolt

1997 "The World's One Hope." In *Bertolt Brecht: Poems 1913-1956*. John Willett and Ralph Manheim, eds. New York: Methuen.

Brinkman, Uwe K.

1991 *The AIDS Epidemic in Thailand*. Boston: Harvard School of Public Health.

Brooks, Peter

1984 *Reading for the Plot: Design and Intention in Narrative*. Cambridge: Harvard University Press.

1994 *Psychoanalysis and Storytelling*. Cambridge: Blackwell Publishers.

Bruner, Jerome

1986 *Actual Minds, Possible Worlds*. Cambridge: Harvard University Press.

1990 *Acts of Meaning*. Cambridge: Harvard University Press.

2004 "Life as Narrative." *Social Research* 71(3):691–710.

Cash, Kathleen

2011 "What's Shame Got to Do With It: Forced Sex among Married and Steady Partners in Uganda," *African Journal of Reproductive Health* 15:25–40.

Cash, Kathleen, Bupa Anasuchatkul, and Wantana Busayawong

1995 *Experimental Educational Interventions for AIDS Prevention among Northern Thai Single Migratory Factory Workers*. Research Report Series: Women and AIDS Research Program. Washington, DC: International Center for Research on Women.

1999 "Understanding the Psychosocial Aspects of HIV/AIDS Prevention for Northern Thai Single Adolescent Migratory Women Workers."*Applied Psychology* 48(2):125–37.

Cash, Kathleen, Hashima-e-Nasreen, Ayesha Aziz, Abbas Bhuiya, A. Mushtaque R. Chowdhury, and Sadia Chowdhury

2001 "Without Sex Education: Understanding the Social and Sexual Vulnerabilities of Rural Bengali Youth," *Sex Education* 1(3):219–33.

Centers for Disease Control and Prevention (CDC)

2003 *HIV/AIDS Surveillance Report 2003*. Atlanta, GA: US Dept of Health and Human Services.

2004 *HIV/AIDS among US Women: Minority and Young Women at Continuing Risk*. Atlanta, GA: US Dept of Health and Human Services.

2006 *HIV/AIDS Among African-Americans Fact Sheet*. Atlanta, GA: US Dept of Health and Human Services.

2007 *HIV/AIDS Among Hispanics—United States, 2001-2005*. Atlanta, GA: US Dept of Health and Human Services.

2008 *HIV/AIDS Among Hispanics/Latinos: Factsheet*. Atlanta, GA: Department of Health and Human Services.

Chowdhury, M. R., A. S. M. M. Rahman, and M. Moniruzzaman
1989   "Serological Investigations for Detection of HIV Infection in Bangladesh."
        Bangladesh Armed Forces Medical Journal 13:20–26.

Cohen, Mardge, Catherine Deamant, Susan Barkan, Jean Richardson, Mary Young, Susan
    Holman, Kathryn Anastos, Judith Cohen, and Sandra Melnick
2000   "Domestic violence and childhood sexual abuse in HIV-infected women and
        women at risk for HIV." *American Journal of Public Health* 90(4):560–65.

Cooley, Charles Horton
2006 [1922] *Human Nature and the Social* Order. New Brunswick: Transaction
        Publishers.

Darwin, Charles
1872   *The Expression of Emotion in Men and Animals*. London: John Murray.

Das, Veena
2000   "The Act of Witnessing: Violence, Poisonous Knowledge, and Subjectivity." In
        Violence and Subjectivity. Veena Das, Arthur Kleinman, Mamphela Ramphele,
        and Pamela Reynolds, eds. Pp. 205–25. Berkeley: University of California Press.

Denizet-Lewis, Benoit
2003   "Double Lives on the Down Low." *New York Times Sunday Magazine*. August 3.

Denzin, Norman K.
1997   "Performance Text," In *Representation and the Text*. William G. Tierney and
        Yvonna S. Lincoln, eds. Pp. 179–218. Albany: State University of New York
        Press.

Deonna, Juliean A., Raffaele Rodogno, and Fabrice Teroni
2012   *In Defense of Shame: The Faces of an Emotion*. New York: Oxford University
        Press.

Dolan, Chris
2009   *Social Torture: The Case of Northern Uganda, 1986–2006*. New York: Berghahm
        Books.

Douglas, Mary
1990 [1950] "Foreward." In *The Gift*, by Marcel Mauss. New York: Routledge.

Farmer, Paul
2003   *Pathologies of Power: Health, Human Rights, and the New War on the Poor*
        California Series in Public Anthropology. Berkeley: University of California
        Press.
2006   *AIDS and Accusation: Haiti and the Geography of Blame*, updated with a new
        preface. Berkeley: University of California Press.

Fassin, Didier
2007   *When Bodies Remember: Experiences and Politics of AIDS in South Africa*.
        Berkeley: University of California Press.
2012   *Humanitarian Reason: A Moral History of the Present*. Berkeley: University of
        California Press.

Finnstrom, Sverker
2008   *Living with Bad Surroundings*. Durham: Duke University Press.

Fishbein, Martin, Susan E. Middlestadt, and Penelope J. Hitchcock

    1991   "Using Information to Change Sexually Transmitted Disease-Related Behaviors: An Analysis Based on the Theory of Reasoned Action." In *Research Issues in Human Behavior and Sexually Transmitted Diseases in the AIDS Era*. Judith Wasserheit, Sevgi O. Aral, and King K. Holmes, eds. Pp. 243–57. Washington, DC: American Society for Microbiology.

Ford, Nicholas, and S. Kittisuksathit

    1994   "Destinations Unknown: The Gender Construction and Changing Nature of the Sexual Lifestyles of Thai Youth." *AIDS Care* 6(5):517–31.

Foucault, Michael

    1980   *Power/Knowledge: Selected Interviews and Other Writings 1972-1977*. Colin Gordon, ed. New York: Pantheon.

Frank, Arthur

    1995   *The Wounded Storyteller: Body, Illness and Ethics*. Chicago: University of Chicago Press.

Freire, Paulo

    1973   *Education for Critical Consciousness*. New York: The Seabury Press.

Fullilove, M. T., R. E. Fullilove III, K. Haynes, and S. Gross

    1990   "Black Women and AIDS Prevention: A View Towards Understanding Gender Rules." *Journal of Sex Research* 27(1):47–64.

Gatrell, V. A. C.

    1994   *The Hanging Tree: Execution and the English People 1770–1868*. Oxford University Press: Oxford.

Geertz, Clifford

    1973   *The Interpretation of Cultures*. New York: Basic Books.

Giddens, Anthony

    1991   *Modernity and Self-Identity: Self and Society in the Late Modern Age*. Redwood City, CA: Stanford University Press.

    1992   *The Transformation of Intimacy: Sexuality, Love, and Eroticism in Modern Societies*. Redwood City, CA: Stanford University Press.

Goffman, Erving

    1959   *The Presentation of Self in Everyday Life*. New York: Anchor Books.

Holquist, Michael

    1990   *Dialogism: Bakhtin and His World*. London: Routledge.

Hussain, M. A., G. S. Rahman, N. G. Banik, and N. Begum

    1996   *A Study to Determine the Prevalence of RTI/STDs in a Rural Area of Bangladesh*. Dhaka: Save the Children USA.

Jackson, Michael

    2002   *The Politics of Storytelling: Violence, Transgression, and Intersubjectivity*. Copenhagen, Denmark: Museum Tusculanum Press.

Kleinman, Arthur

    1988   *The Illness Narratives: Suffering, Healing, and the Human Condition*. New York: Basic Books

Kleinman, Arthur, and Erin Fitz-Henry

2007   "The Experiential Basis of Subjectivity: How Individuals Change in the Context
of Societal Transformation." In *Subjectivity: Ethnographic Investigations*. Biehl
Joao, Byron Good, and Arthur Kleinman, eds. Pp. 52–65. Berkeley: University
of California Press.

Langer, Lawrence L.

1997   "The Alarmed Vision: Social Suffering and Holocaust Atrocity." In *Social
Suffering*. Arthur Kleinman, Veena Das and Margaret Lock, eds. Pp. 47–66.
Berkeley: University of California Press.

Lara, Maria Pia

2007   *Narrating Evil: A Postmetaphysical Theory of Reflective Judgment*. New York:
Columbia University Press.

Levi, Primo

1959   *If This is a Man*. New York: Orion Press.

1988   *Collected Poems*. London: Faber and Faber.

1989   *The Drowned and the Saved*. New York: Vintage International.

Levinas, Emmanuel

2003 [1935]   *On Escape: De l'évasion* (*Cultural Memory in the Present*). Bettina Bergo,
trans. Redwood City, CA: Stanford University Press.

Lewis, Helen

1971   *Shame and Guilt in Neurosis*. New York: International Universities Press.

Lewis, Laurence A., and William J. Coffey

1985   "The Continuing Deforestation of Haiti." *Ambio* 14(3):158–60.

Lewis-Williams, David

2002   *The Mind in the Cave*. London: Thames & Hudson, Ltd.

Lichtenstein, Bronwen

2004   "Domestic Violence, Sexual Ownership, and HIV Risk in Women in the
American Deep South." *Social Science & Medicine* 60(4):701–14.

Mahoney-Anderson, P. J., A. Wohl, and M. Yu-Harlan

2000   *An Epidemiologic Profile of HIV and AIDs in Los Angeles County*. Los Angeles:
LAC Department of Health Services.

Marushak, L. M.

2002   *HIV in Prisons 2000*. Publication No. NCJ-196023L US Department of Justice,
Office of Justice Programs, Bureau of Justice Statistics. Washington, DC: US
Government Printing Office.

Maticka-Tyndale, Eleanor, Melissa Haswell-Elkins, Thicumporn Kuyyakanond, Monthira
Kiewying, and David Elkins

1994   "A Research-Based HIV Intervention in Northeast Thailand." Supplement to
Volume 4, AIDS Impact and Prevention: Demographic and Social Science
Perspectives. *Health Transition Review* 4(Suppl):349–67.

Mattingly, Cheryl

1998   *Healing Dramas and Clinical Plots: The Narrative Structure of Experience*.
Cambridge: Cambridge University Press.

Mattingly, Cheryl, and Linda C. Garro
   2000   "Narrative as Construct and Construction." In *Narrative and the Cultural Construction of Illness and Healing*. Cheryl Mattingly and Linda C. Garro, eds. Pp. 1–49. Berkeley: University of California Press.

Mauss, Marcel
   1990 [1950] *The Gift*. Abingdon, Oxon: Routledge.

Miller, Jacques-Alain
   2006   "On Shame." In *Jacques Lacan and the Other Side of Psychoanalysis: Reflections on Seminar XVII*. Justin Clemens and Russell Grigg, eds. Pp. 1–11. Durham: Duke University Press.

Mitra, S. N., A. Al-Sabir, and A. R. Cross
   1997   *Bangladesh: Demographic and Health Survey 1996–1997*. Dhaka, Bangladesh, and Calverton, MD: National Institute of Population Research and Training (NIPORT), Mitra and Associates, and Macro International Inc.

Moreau, Ron
   1992   "Sex and Death in Thailand." *Newsweek* 120(3):50–51.

Morgan, Michael
   2008   *On Shame*. New York: Routledge.

Murray, Gerald F., and Glen R. Smucker
   2004   *The Uses of Children: Trafficking Haitian Children*. Port au Prince, Haiti: USAID/Haiti Mission.

Nietzsche, Friedrich
   2007 [1886] *On the Genealogy of Morality*. New York: Vintage.

Ochs, Elinor, and Lisa Capps
   1996   "Narrating the Self." *Annual Review of Anthropology* 25:19–43.

Plummer, Ken
   1995   *Telling Sexual Stories: Power, Change and Social Worlds*. London: Routledge.

Probyn, Elspeth
   2005   *Blush: Faces of Shame*. Minneapolis: University of Minnesota Press.

Pulerwitz, Julie, Steven L. Gortmaker, and William DeJong
   2000   "Measuring Sexual Relationship Power in HIV/STD Research." *Sex Roles* 42(7-8):637–60.

Pyne, Hnin Hnin
   1992   *AIDS and Prostitution in Thailand: A Case Study of Burmese Prostitutes in Ranong*. Master's Thesis, Department of Urban Studies and Planning, Massachusetts Institute of Technology.

Ratner, M. S., ed.
   1993   *Crack Pipe as Pimp: An Ethnographic Investigation of Sex-for-Crack Exchanges*. New York: Lexington Books.

Reback, Cathy J., Paul A. Simon, Cathleen C. Bemis, and Bobby Gatson
   2001   *The Los Angeles Transgender Health Study: Community Report*. Dr. Cathy J. Reback (Rbackcj@aol.com). Funded by the Universitywide AIDS Research Program, University of California grant number #PC97-LAC-012I.. Additional

funding provided by the California State Office of AIDS and the County of Los Angeles, Department of Health Services, Office of AIDS Programs and Policy.

Rosenstock, Irwin M.

1974   "Historical Origins of the Health Belief Model." *Health Education Behavior* 2(4):328–35.

Rosenstock, Irwin M., Victor J. Stecher, and Marshall H. Becker

1994   "The Health Belief Model and HIV Behavior Risk." *Preventing AIDS: Theories and Methods of Behavioral Interventions*. R. J. DiClemente and John L. Peterson, eds. Pp. 5–24. New York: Plenum Press.

Scheff, Thomas J.

2003   "Shame in Self and Society." *Symbolic Interaction* 26(2):239–62.

Scheff, Thomas J., and Suzanne M. Retzinger

1991   *Emotions and Violence: Shame and Rage in Destructive Conflicts*. Massachusetts: Lexington Books.

Scheper-Hughes, Nancy

2007   "Violence and the Politics of Remorse: Lessons from South Africa." In *Subjectivity: Ethnographic Investigations*. Joao Biehl, Byron Good, and Arthur Kleinman, eds. Pp. 179–324. Berkeley: University of California Press.

Scheub, Harold

2006   *Storytelling Songs of Zulu Women*. Lewiston: The Edwin Mellen Press.

Scott, James C.

1990   *Domination and the Arts of Resistance*. New Haven: Yale University Press.

Sen, Amartya

1999   *Development as Freedom*. Anchor Books: New York.

Sharf, Barbara F., and Marsha L. Vanderford

2003   "Illness Narratives and the Social Construction of Health." In *Handbook of Health Communication*. Teresa L. Thompson, Alicia Dorsey, and Katherine Miller, eds. Pp. 9–34. Mahwah, NJ: Routledge.

Smith, Jennie.

2001   *When the Hands are Many*. Ithaca: Cornell University Press.

Sontag, Susan

2003   *Regarding the Pain of Others*. New York: Farrar, Straus and Giroux.

Tangney, J. P., and R. L. Dearing

2002   *Shame and Guilt*. New York: The Guilford Press.

Tarakeshwar, N., A. Fox, C. Ferro, S. Khawaja, A. Kochman, and K.J. Sikkema

2005   "The Connections Between Childhood Sexual Abuse and Human Immunodeficiency Virus Infection: Implications for Interventions." *Journal of Community Psychology* 33(6):655–72.

Taylor, Charles

1985   "The Person." In *The Category of the Person: Anthropology, Philosophy, History*. Michael Carrithers, Steven Collins and Steven Lukes, eds. Pp. 257–81. Cambridge: Cambridge University Press.

Uganda Ministry of Health

2011   *Uganda AIDS Indicator Survey* (UAIS). Kampala: Uganda Ministry of Health.

Valdiserri, Ronald O.
    1989   *Preventing AIDS: The Design of Effective Programs.* New Brunswick, NJ: Rutgers
            University Press.
Wa Mungai, Mbugua, and David A. Samper
    2006   "'No Mercy, No Remorse': Personal Experience Narratives about Public
            Passenger Transportation in Nairobi, Kenya." *Africa Today* 52(3):51–81.
Weniger, Bruce, K. Limpakarnjanarat, K. Ungchusak, S. Thanprasertsuk, K. Choopanya,
    S. Vanichseni, T. Uneklabh, P. Thongcharoen, and W. Chantapong
    1991   "The Epidemiology of HIV Infection and AIDS in Thailand." *AIDS* 5(Suppl
            2):571–85.
Williams, Bernard.
    1993   *Shame and Necessity.* Berkeley: University of California Press.
Wohl, A.R., S. Lu, S. Odem, F. Sorvillo, C.F. Pegues, and P. R. Kerndt
    1998   "Sociodemographic and Behavioral Characteristics of African-American Women
            with HIV and AIDS in Los Angeles County 1990–1997." *Journal of Acquired
            Immune Deficiency Syndromes* 19(4):413–20.
Wollheim, Richard
    1999   *On the Emotions.* New Haven: Yale University Press.
World Bank
    2007   *Social Resilience and State Fragility in Haiti.* The World Bank Report Country
            Study. Washington, DC: The World Bank.
World Health Organization
    1998   *UNAIDS/WHO Working Group on Global HIV/AIDS and STD Surveillance.*
            Geneva: WHO Global HIV/AIDS and STD Surveillance Program.
    2003   *The World Health Report 2003: Shaping the Future.* Geneva: World Health
            Organization.
Worth, Dooley
    1989   "Sexual Decision-Making and AIDS: Why Condom Promotion Among
            Vulnerable Women is Likely to Fail." *Studies in Family Planning* 20(6):297–307.
Yea, Sallie
    2005   "Labour of Love: Filipina Entertainer's Narratives of Romance and
            Relationships with GI in US Military Camp Towns in Korea." *Women's Studies
            International Forum* 28(6):456–72.

Index